# ENDORSEMENTS

"Arrrrrr... Captain, well done sir! I salute lucid dreaming and the evolution of your lingo."—Mr. Pat Desjardins, Chief Petty Officer (retired), Royal Canadian Navy, Victoria, BC, Canada.

"I read your last book: it was unconventional, surprisingly beautiful, and I hear this one's the masterpiece."—Mr. Paul Hix, Building Maintenance Engineer, Victoria, BC, Canada.

"Absolutely brilliant! I encourage all the dreamers in the world to read this book because it proves we all have a deeper power within us."—Ms Karen O'Meara, School Teacher/Counsellor (retired), Victoria, BC, Canada.

"Thanks for your seventh book about lucid dreaming – no review could ever do justice to the valuable views and incredible ideas inside these amazing paperbacks!"—Mr. Martin Schicci, Electrician and Supervisor of the Electrical Department at the Royal Jubilee Hospital in Victoria, BC, Canada.

"Captivating, uplifting, and fun to read... propelled by fast paced revelations from a lucid dreamer who describes a meaningful point to life!" ––Mr. Steve Smith, Chief Engineer of the power plant at the Royal Jubilee Hospital in Victoria, BC, Canada.

# HEALTHY DREAMS, HAPPY LIFE

Written by "Captain"
## WILLIAM MOFFAT
Power Engineer and Master of Clinical Hypnotherapy

Healthy Dreams, Happy Life
Copyright © 2020 by William Moffat

All rights reserved. No part of this publication may be reproduced, distributed, or transmitted in any form or by any means, including photocopying, recording, or other electronic or mechanical methods, without the prior written permission of the author, except in the case of brief quotations embodied in critical reviews and certain other non-commercial uses permitted by copyright law.

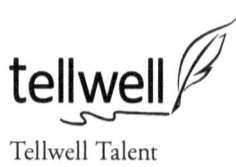

Tellwell Talent
www.tellwell.ca

ISBN
978-0-2288-4164-7 (Paperback)

Dedicated to…

A pop song –
<u>Return From Failure</u> – by William Moffat

and with
gratitude to
Patty "High Pockets",
Karen O'Meara, and Ann Moffat
for their input!

# HEALTHY DREAMS, HAPPY LIFE

Lucid dreaming is incredible! That's because while you're sleeping, a different level of your self-awareness can bring a lucid dream world to life. Lucid awareness is a conscious viewpoint causing you to realize that you're in a dream world.

Questioning the meaning of lucid dreams parallels another ancient query: "What's the meaning of life?" Healthy lucid dreaming explains how and why – by balancing conscious and subconscious energy – healthy happiness can be brought to life.

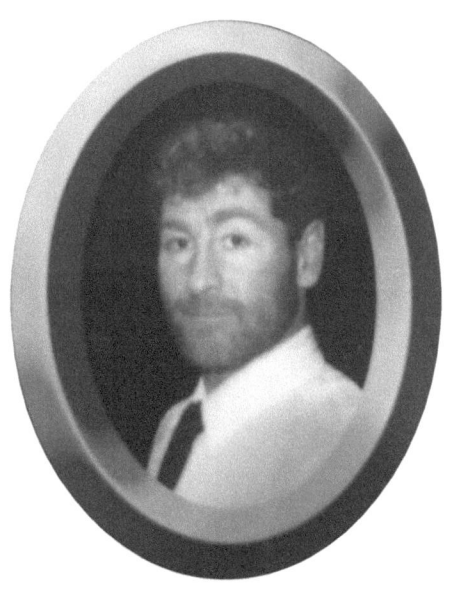

# ABOUT THE WRITER – "CAPTAIN" WILLIAM MOFFAT

I love living in Victoria, on Vancouver Island, British Columbia, Canada, where I work as a Power Engineer. My nickname is "Captain" because long ago, I was an officer cadet at Royal Roads Military College in Victoria – decades after my honourable discharge, I'm still getting called "Captain" by some civilian and military friends.

From officer cadet to "Captain", I've been involved with various fields of study, mixed occupations, and have travelled the world. Nowadays, unless I'm working, sleeping, or writing, you may find me strumming a guitar on the beach below my downtown condominium.

# TABLE OF CONTENTS

**Chapter 1   A Deep Step Into Lucid Dreaming** .................................. 1
   The Motorcycle Lucid Dream ........................................... 4
   Profound Insight ................................................................ 6
   The Earthy Lucid Dream ................................................. 11
   Transformative Steps ...................................................... 14
   The Tropical Beach Lucid Dream ................................... 16
   A Soul Saving Lucid Dream ............................................ 19

**Chapter 2   A Step Further** ............................................................... 23
   Reflections ....................................................................... 26
   The Fighter Pilot Lucid Dream ....................................... 27
   An Especially Special Erotic Lucid Dream .................... 29
   The Recurring Nightmares ............................................. 32
   The Clincher Lucid Dream ............................................. 37

**Chapter 3   Dream Reviews and Revelations** .................................. 43
   The Albatross Lucid Dream ............................................ 45
   Lucid Awareness .............................................................. 47
   Front To Back Thinking (FTBT) ................................... 51

**Chapter 4   The Dreamer** .................................................................. 55
   The Golden Lucid Dream ............................................... 58
   Glorious Wonder! ........................................................... 64
   Ego Consciousness .......................................................... 67
   Ego, And Egotism ........................................................... 70
   Taking A New Path ......................................................... 71
   Good, And Evil ............................................................... 73

**Chapter 5   Eternity And The Moment** ........................................... 76
   Space ................................................................................ 82
   The Essence Of Self-awareness ....................................... 83
   Time ................................................................................. 84
   Aligning With Deeper Self-awareness ............................ 88
   Strain Due To A Lack Of Stress ...................................... 90
   The Nemesis Of Ultimate Enlightenment ..................... 92
   Another Step Toward Loving The Mystery Of Death ... 94

**Chapter 6  Death's Door** ...........................................................96
   A Fear Of Death ................................................................. 99
   The Thunderbird Lucid Dream ..................................... 100
   An Alert! ............................................................................103
   Re-Birth ............................................................................ 106
   Reincarnation .................................................................. 109
   Original Human Consciousness ...................................... 111

**Chapter 7  You're Not Superior to Anyone; No Way!** ............ 115
   Aggressive Surprise ...........................................................116
   Happy Life ........................................................................118
   A Paradox of Self-awareness ........................................... 120
   A Truer Meaning Of Happiness ..................................... 122

**Chapter 8  Freedom From Fear of Fear** ................................ 127
   Firewalker ........................................................................ 136

**Chapter 9  Conscious and Subconscious Balance** .................. 140
   Useful ................................................................................141
   Thankful .......................................................................... 144
   Respectful ........................................................................ 146
   Healthy .............................................................................147
   The Angel Lucid Dream ................................................. 148
   Compassionate ................................................................ 153
   Forgiveness For Fearful Feedback ....................................154
   Trustful ............................................................................ 157

**Chapter 10  A Quick Review Of Lucid Law** ........................ 160
   The Lucid Law Of Love ...................................................161
   The Lucid Law Of Resistance ..........................................163
   The Lucid Boomerang Law .............................................165
   The Lucid Law Of Forgiveness ........................................167
   The Lucid Law Of Belief ................................................ 168
   The Lucid Law Of Living In The Now ..........................170
   The Lucid Law Of Tossing Your Burden .......................172
   A Fun-loving Finish! ........................................................173

# CHAPTER ONE

# A DEEP STEP INTO LUCID DREAMING

Because different levels of self-awareness bring different types of dream worlds to life, insight into healthy, and disturbing dream worlds can be really fun! Lots of folks want to know what their dreams mean. For example: early one morning, a young woman smiled at her husband and said, "I just dreamt that you gave me a pretty pearl necklace for my birthday. Everything seemed so real. What do you think such a dream could mean?"

"Sweetheart, you'll know tonight," he answered – with his own dreamy smile.

That evening, the husband came home with a small package wrapped in ribbons and bows. He called out, "Happy birthday babe!"

Merrily, she opened the promising looking gift. Her jaw suddenly dropped. He'd given her a book, Pearls Of Wisdom From Lucid Dreaming. She snorted with muffled laughter and said, "Thanks for the pearls."

Some people may become lucidly aware while asleep and dreaming. For me, having lucid awareness is like being in the real world, but I know I'm in a different dimension of reality while a lucid dream is happening. So for you, checking out a few of my most pivotal lucid dreams can be a healthy way to discover some proven pearls of wisdom pouring from a deeper meaning of lucid dream life. This way, having had your own lucid dream isn't central since simply agreeing that you've had any sort of a dream – while sleeping – is a start. So c'mon, it's time to have some fun!

Decades ago, I began recording my dream experiences. I've been paying attention to psychologically healthy – sometimes psychologically unhealthy – dream worlds by jotting down notes in dream diaries. Since I'm a passionate writer, quite a few big boxes have filled with my dream diaries. That's why there's plenty for me to talk about.

After waking up, most folks can remember having been in a dream world. Generally, while asleep and dreaming, people don't realize they're in a different dimension of reality; lucid dreaming is different. Lucid dreaming is all about realizing I'm dreaming while the dream is happening. While at a lucid level of self-awareness, I love the way the dream world seems so real. That's because I believe that such a world is made from subconscious energy. The "idea" that subconscious energy can appear and feel like a physical reality never ceases to amaze me!

Even though I'll usually have only one, there're times when I can "live" through several lucid dreams in one night; however, sometimes months may go by without any at all. Realization of being in a dream world (later in my life I learned it was called lucid dreaming) didn't seem odd until my early teens. Discussion about dreaming, with fellow classmates, revealed that no one else ever realized they were in a dream fantasy while the fantasy was happening.

Banging my head (in just the right spot) against a wall during my early childhood could be responsible for the way I seem to suddenly awaken from sleep – while still in a dream world. Instead of banging your head against a wall, starting a dream diary is a healthier way to go! That's because getting more familiar with your dream worlds helps you to recognize when you're in one.

A daily diary helps a person recall main events that happened in the real world. Also, merely writing down whatever you believe was happening can put experiences into fresh perspective. A dream diary helps a person recall dream world experiences, and just writing down whatever you thought was happening can bring new perspective on dream life. Plus, getting good at remembering dreams makes "living" your own lucid dream a real possibility.

In order to always remember a dream, I keep a closed notebook – with a pencil stowed inside – under my pillow. The instant I awaken from sleep, I can open this book to write brief notes about my dream life. Leaving the lights off makes getting back to sleep a lot easier. Later, after my sleep period, especially if the dream was a lucid one, I'll often add a more readable account – a report with good detail.

If you're clever enough to own a cell phone, you might take advantage of a built in voice recorder, eventually transferring the recordings to a computer file, or a stand alone recorder can be used. There's tremendous benefit from journaling these testimonies because after reviewing them, you're capable of becoming well acquainted with dreaming. Being more familiar with your dream life makes remembering your real-life identity – while dreaming – a lot easier.

There's a possibility for you to link with your own deeper dreaming self – the "One" who you believe you are in the real world – by merging with a level of lucid awareness while dreaming. Lucid awareness during a dream world might sound strange since the fabric for any dream world arrives from the subconscious mind. In fact, a person's subconscious mind can be so powerful that it may be called multidimensional since it's capable of powering up new dimensions of dream reality!

A person can believe that a dream world is real-life reality – while the dream is happening – because they're not fully awake. Although dream life might seem weird, unfamiliar, or disturbing, any type of dream world can feel perfectly real. The same as remembering real-world experiences, people usually remember dream experiences from one point of view, as though being a separate self. That's why a dream diary is usually written from an individual point of view, same as the way a typical real-world diary is composed.

From a deeper perspective, the dreamer is every individual dream character – all at the same time. If one of the individual dream characters merges with the dreamer's belief in self-definition, then a memory of real-life reality gets channelled into that one individual. This one individual's level of self-awareness transforms into lucid awareness – a presence of mind who's consciously aware that they're dreaming.

For me, a lucid dream only ever has one lucidly aware presence of mind taking place at a time. If the transformation into lucid awareness happens for a dream character who isn't human, but perhaps is in the form of a bird for example, then that one living dream "entity" attains lucid awareness, and I realize I'm in a dream world!

Shortly after I turned twenty-one, a lucid dream motivated me to begin keeping a dream diary. At the beginning of this motivational lucid dream, I was riding a motorcycle along a mountain highway. Suddenly, I became lucid, understood that I was in a dream! While riding that motorcycle, I realized I was really at home, safe in my bed, sound asleep!

## The Motorcycle Lucid Dream

Absolutely certain that I was in a dream fantasy, an idea caught my attention. Because the motorcycle seemed to be exactly the same as the one I rode in real life, here was a chance to discover my bike's limits while going through a curve in the highway. That's why I decided to keep accelerating until I wiped-out! Since I was in a dream world, I wouldn't be killed by the crash. I felt immortal while in the dream world because I trusted – no matter what happened – I would eventually reawaken into my real-world reality.

All of my attention was focused on the road in front of me. My right hand automatically rolled the throttle grip – the engine blasted, the big street bike accelerated. While picking up speed, I leaned the heavy motorcycle to the right, right into an upcoming curve. My motorbike was tilted at such a steep angle that a chrome exhaust pipe brushed the pavement. Even though the day was sunny and bright, in my peripheral vision I could see red hot sparks showering out beneath me. Clearly, I wouldn't be making it past this bend.

I felt a little disappointed with my motorbike because a glance at the speedometer proved this wasn't going to be the super high-speed performance I was anticipating. Plus, I treasured my big beautiful street bike, cringed at the thought of losing control.

Anguish suddenly gave way to an unexpected searing pain from a lower limb: my right leg had become trapped between the pavement and sliding bike! The moment was intensely real and the excruciating pain was alarming – I knew this was all a dream, so why did my leg hurt so much?

Since the rear wheel was free from the road, the over-revving engine roared, and as pain ravaged one side of my body I thought: "Wow, so this is how it feels to wipe-out!"

The lucid dream fantasy kept going… there was a weird sensation of weightlessness followed by a heavy G-force as my motorcycle and I flipped and tumbled over a gravel embankment. I landed in a deep ditch full of thorny blackberry bushes, the big bike crashing down on top of me. The engine had died, there was an eerie silence mixed with dust filled air, and I felt astounded by how real everything seemed!

Although my head could move a little, the rest of me was seriously injured. With my dream body torn and broken, I felt like a life-size rag doll that'd been tossed, ripped to shreds, and then pinned into a shadowy ditch. As dust settled, I noticed a few flickering rays of sunshine sifting through the great gash in the mass of bushy thorns which had clawed up my leather jacket, pants, and me on the way in. Finally, a stinging pain coming from fiery droplets of multihued gasoline dripping over my wounds combined with the smell of burning flesh. I did not like the way things were going! My lucid dream fantasy had become a nightmare and the thought of being burned to death made me want to wake up. Suddenly, I realized that I was awake!

While contorted like a pretzel, with one arm bent around the back of one of my ruined legs, a subconscious urge caused me to pinch myself on the back of the leg as hard as possible – and at the same time, twist the flesh where I was pinching. I pinched and twisted my skin severely – I wanted to return home! The odd sense of dull numbness taking place where I was pinching and twisting immediately turned into an intense form of ticklish pain. At last, there was a sudden jolt, and I was back home in my bed, still wide awake!

I felt a huge relief to be back in my bed; a freedom which eventually faded after my grasping the truth that I'd never really been gone. While checking over my pain-free body with anxious hands, I was totally stunned. My motorcycle crash experience seemed absolutely authentic, yet, here I was safe and sound with no broken bones, burns, bruises, or cuts. There was definitely something different about that dream, and I knew there'd been many others over the years which shared the quality of such realism, but my memory of their details was hazy. I understood how a few hints could bring me a flood of memories. That's why the idea to start a dream diary hit me like a ton of bricks – recordings could give me the hints I needed to always remember the dream.

Feeling so shaken and moved by my motorcycle crash nightmare, I hopped out of bed and searched for a pencil and some paper to write down clear notes while the dream was still fresh in my memory. Right then and there, I made a solemn promise to continue writing about my dream experiences. After finding an unused notebook (it fit perfectly under my pillow), my first dream diary took form.

The next morning, while reading through my dream diary's notes, I understood why a severe pinch and twist of the skin was something important to remember. To this day, the feeling I get from an especially light pinch lets me know if I'm dreaming or if I'm in the real world. A light pinch followed by instant pain means I'm definitely here in real-life reality. What's more, a light pinch of the skin on any part of my body, along with my feeling a strange sensation of dull numbness, tells me I'm in a dream. This way, I can escape from a nightmare since a really hard pinch and twist jolts me back home. To be clear, although this especially light pinch test feels strangely numb while I'm in a lucid dream, any other sense of touch feels the same as when I'm in the real world.

Throughout my life, I've been performing the pinch test to double-check on where I am because dreamlike stuff can occur in the real world… like the time when I experienced a mild earthquake. At first, I didn't understand what was happening; however, a quick pinch on my rear produced sharp pain… so, at least I knew I was in real-life reality!

I trust that the real-life "me" can't really be killed by what happens in a lucid dream. That's because I consciously believe that I'll eventually return home. For me, lucid awareness during a lucid dream tosses any fear of death; nevertheless, a fear of pain stays!

## **Profound Insight**

Capable of a lot more than just powering up physical sensation, subconscious power can also numb part or all of a person's body. In addition, such subconscious power doesn't have to come from conscious fear! Some dentists and doctors take advantage of hypnotic techniques to perform pain free operations without the use of anaesthetics on their more trusting patients. What's more, after gaining a sense of rapport with an amputee, a hypnotherapist can use hypnosis to eliminate phantom pain felt in the amputated limb's extremities – real pain that may linger long after the person's limb was amputated.

A person's mind is actually a combination of conscious and subconscious energy. Although consciousness does all the thinking, the subconscious experiences an awareness of physical sensation, and emotion. A person's conscious belief impresses their subconscious mind, and the subconscious part of their mind impresses the conscious part with physical and emotional feelings. This way, a presence of mind can feel real.

My mind has imagined so many dream worlds that just thinking about trying to record them all feels monumental; meanwhile, ever since my <u>Motorcycle</u> lucid dream took place, as long as I've pencil and paper at hand, I'll always jot down a few notes about lucid dreaming. Such notes have helped me gain deeper subconscious power to manage the way my subconscious energy streams forth, yet, my learning curve had (and still has) some big dips.

One of my biggest backward thinking dips took place due to an epiphany! While rereading through my first dream diary, I noticed that my lucid dreams had a common link – since I'd always be so caught up with the realness and magnitude of a lucid dream world, I wouldn't even consider the profoundness of why everything was happening.

After reviewing more and more dream diary data, I began to believe that all dream worlds were miracles of creation because these different dimensions of reality came into existence by means of conscious and subconscious energy interacting. A lucid dream world seemed most miraculous because being able to live out my most intimate sexual desires during these types of fantasies finally dawned on me. I was a tall, skinny (and single) twenty-four year old; the summer morning was bright, but my epiphany was even brighter!

Frustration arrived in a roundabout way. That's because after feeling the odd sensation of dull numbness coming from my gentle pinch, I'd completely focus on experiencing a different dimension of what seemed like my real-world reality; however, in this dimension of existence, I could have a seemingly real sexual encounter with a beautiful woman!

Exhilaration accompanying such sudden realization would blow the top off my conscious mind, and I'd return home pre-maturely.

Quite often, months can go by without my having any lucid dreams. That's why it took several years for me to figure out how to make my new, deeper thinking lucid awareness last longer. For me, deeper thinking lucid awareness is all about understanding how to balance conscious and subconscious energy while dreaming. Throughout this period of my life, merging with a level of lucid awareness made me experience a rush of powerful exhilaration; then, I'd automatically jolt back home all too soon.

Entries in my dream diary kept reminding me about my lucid dreaming, and these reminders helped cultivate some lucid dream survival techniques. Later on in life, the notes about basic rules and techniques to make lucid dreams last longer would lead to seven supporting ideas and understandings that I've dubbed as being "Lucid Law".

My seven lucid laws have become useful for guiding the way a lucid dream world unfolds, and they've deep parallels in the real world. You're capable of gaining a whole new perspective on the meaning of dreaming and on a truer meaning of life if you can understand these new ideas. Right off the bat, you can begin to play with the notion that during any dream world, a multidimensional mind creates and lives a whole new space-time continuum! A dream world's space continuum is subconscious energy at work while the time continuum is conscious energy at play. In other words, a dream world's present moment is consciously and subconsciously self-aware. Longer lasting lucid awareness during a lucid dream world makes the new dimension of reality last longer.

The seven lucid dream laws help keep my lucid level of self-awareness energized, and my lucid dreaming lasts longer. Understanding Lucid Law provides a clear path into incredible subconscious power for the lucid dreamer. Having control over my own subconscious mind gets my lucidly aware dream character some astonishing power to play with because during a lucid dream world, subconscious energy can create anything my conscious mind can imagine. Gaining control over my conscious mind's imagination and command over deeper subconscious power to direct the way a lucid dream world unfolds is what Lucid Law is really about. That's why lucid awareness makes me realize that my time in a lucid dream world has the potential to be the time of my life!

In those early years of discovery, I seemed to be taking two steps backward for each step forward. I kept going down this front to back thinking path and eventually experienced longer lasting lucid dreams! Although I felt like I was going backwards, sometimes upside-down, and even inside-out, I continued to write (and reread) in my dream diary.

Seeming to take forever, there was finally one special morning that brought new insight – an eye opener that would help make my lucid dreaming last longer. My revelation came from an especially clear note in my dream diary: it was about finding direction, and this suggestion led to an exciting epiphany about keeping a lucid dream world alive. That morning, a new realization dawned on me: I'd been going in the wrong real-life direction; to step deeper into lucid dreaming, turning my real life around was the correct direction I really needed to go in!

Stepping away from my own selfish outlooks on being the proud and impressive person who I honestly believed I was supposed to be here in the real world brought forward a new attitude, one really important pearl of wisdom pouring from my short-lived lucid dreams – if I could come up with a deeper-thinking concept of self-definition in the real world, then maybe my lucid awareness could last longer in a lucid dream world. That's why I began to take a closer look at who I wanted to be compared to who I really was – I wanted to be happy, but I really wasn't.

Thanks to new insight arriving from my dream diary, the underlying unhappiness I felt from unhealthy truth behind some of my real-life beliefs began to come clear. For instance: if I felt proud to be a man, was I believing that my consciousness was superior due to my male gender? In my dream worlds, gender didn't make my dream character superior or inferior – a belief in being alive made my dream character feel important!

I began to understand why conscious belief in who I am in the real world needed a change in direction in order to make my deeper thinking level of lucid awareness last longer. Maybe I'd be happier if I could learn to be less of a stuffed shirt, less strategic and formal? Because I felt so much excitement about being free from self-centered and egotistical outlooks while in a lucid dream, my new belief in self-definition was overwhelming. This fantastic idea of taking self-definition in a whole new direction was causing me to jolt back home way too soon!

Since the lucid awareness taking place during a lucid dream is my real-life presence of mind, I grasped hold of the notion that I could test a different, deeper thinking direction in my real world. In order to be the one who I wanted to be instead of the one who I was supposed to be, I came up with an innovative plan: a different level of self-definition could be explored from a deeper thinking, real-life outlook. I wanted to go in the opposite direction of having to behave like a properly programmed and superficially superior robot all the time – this monkey wanted to dance and play!

An intention to change my unhealthy real-life outlook began to take a hold of me because I was starting to understand why a healthier outlook during a lucid dream could make healthy happiness last longer. A caring attitude could make any dream unfold in a really good way, while an attitude filled with selfish pride and a greedy desire to feel superior could energize a nightmare! This contrary and backward stepping approach opened a new path for me because I recognized corresponding effects coming from attitudes in the real world. Depending on attitudes, a real-life outlook can also feel good or bad!

A desire to feel good added momentum for my "front to back" stepping direction in the real world since another new idea finally dawned on me: a healthier attitude would make any dimension of reality feel way more fun! A heart beating good mood was what I really wanted to have last longer. That's why my recordings of these brilliant bursts of lucid awareness taking place in the short-lived lucid dream worlds continued in earnest.

I was eventually able to look at the brief lucid dream diary entries in a more scientific way by asking myself questions such as: "In any type of dream, or in the real world, what in the world were attitudes really all about and why were they happening?" I also wondered how and why a dream world could seem so real? Then again, how come the real world seems so real?

After returning home from scores of short-lived lucid dream worlds, I began writing about how the onset of my lucid awareness made me feel as though I'd hold of a genie's magic lamp, but I'd an unlimited amount of wishes at hand! The first wish I wanted to have come true was a calmer attitude at the onset of lucid awareness. Ha! Not so easy to grant such a wish! While they're happening, lucid dream worlds are as believable as any real-life existence. That's why lucid awareness had become short-lived – my conscious belief in the possibility of being able to experience a brief and intense love affair unbalanced my dreaming mind to such a degree that I returned home all too soon.

## The Earthy Lucid Dream

One giant step in a healthy direction for longer lasting lucid awareness took place during an "Earthy" lucid dream. While I was focused on a patch of ground between my bare feet – and enabling a feeling of boredom to slowly sink in – this lucid dream kept going! Focusing all of my attention downward, I got right down on my hands and knees, took a really close look at the grassy ground I was on. Incredibly, lucid dream worlds have the same infinitesimal details as does the real world: bright green blades of grass with tiny intricate roots, pink coloured wiggly worms, lively little ants, moist warm earth, the whole lot.

At first, my view was only a bit boring, but after what seemed like a fairly long time, I began to sink into a deeper state of boredom. Since I was starting to lose the lucid link with my dreaming mind, I intentionally gave one of my butt cheeks a hard pinch and twist, and returned home with that familiar jolt. I wanted to record this emerging discovery in my dream diary as soon as possible. Focusing all of my attention onto the ground between my feet – directly after merging with lucid awareness – would be a good rule to follow at the beginning of every lucid dream. A little boredom could quieten my conscious energy; then, my subconscious energy could keep the dream powered!

During a science class, way back when I was in junior high school, I'd originally learned about this method of grounding overexcited conscious energy – in a healthy way. That's because overflowing with high-spirited teenage energy and some unruly classroom behaviour, a bunch of us students were banished to the school's back lawn; we were tasked with working on a grounding exercise. Ordered to stare into a square foot of turf for twenty minutes, I became more and more intimate with my little patch of grass. The longer I focused on this remarkable world where so much life existed, the deeper I saw into the grass-roots of real-life reality.

When the twenty minutes were up, the science teacher had to come and rouse me – my subconscious mind had become so mesmerized by my conscious focus on the crumbs of commotion going on in my square foot of turf that the twenty minutes flew by. I remember feeling doubly surprised because no one else was as "cool" with the tiny world of bugs and bits of greenery as I was.

Although the rest of the kids got bored right away (and walked away), this exercise helped ground the spirit of unruly teenage excitement; calmer attitudes stepped forward. That's because afterwards, in order to cool down any unruly classroom behaviour, the science teacher only had to suggest another grounding exercise. In retrospect, I think the teacher was wise to try and transform the spirit of teenage excitement into a state of boredom because being bored is a passive, but effective form of self-help for any kid who isn't interested in their school work.

I was reminded of the junior high school grounding exercise after examining the small patch of grassy ground between my feet during the <u>Earthy</u> lucid dream. Since my attention focused deep into the patch of grass, my conscious mind stayed passive, enabling the lucid dream fantasy to keep going for quite a while.

After rereading the dream diary data from my calming <u>Earthy</u> lucid dream, I knew that I could easily gain control over my initial rush of overexcitement during any upcoming lucid dream world. All I had to do was focus on the ground directly between my feet – immediately – at the start of lucid awareness. Finally, my lucid level of self-awareness could last longer! Not only that, I understood why applying this technique for grounding the overexcited spirit of my lucid awareness was similar to following the simpler rules of electrodynamics.

Boredom grounds any unruly spirit of consciousness, enabling the subconscious mind (the "physical" dream world) to continue channelling conscious energy. An underlying rule about the dynamics of lucid awareness is that along with all energy's "physical" realism, conscious energy gets channelled within the dream world's time continuum. That's because there's always a balance of power in play between conscious and subconscious energy. Although self-aware, subconscious energy doesn't actually think. The subconscious mind is automatic, kind of like a computer program. That's why with calmer consciousness there's more boredom and vice versa, with rabble-rousing consciousness there's less boredom. Along with the calmest level of consciousness, a level that has no resistance to boredom, there's deeper connection with the subconscious mind.

For those not-so-scientific-minded folks, I recognized how and why my amazing step into long-lasting lucid dream worlds happened so subtly, through this less resistive approach. It fit with what I later recorded as being the "Lucid Law of Resistance" because when I lowered my resistance to boredom, I calmed my conscious mind enough to stay connected with my subconscious mind. That is, my subconscious dream world could continue channelling calmer consciousness, and keep the lucid dream going!

To call this Lucid Law "resistive" is counterintuitive and requires a reminder of its meaning. The reason why a basic underlying idea behind the Lucid Law of Resistance is about resistance instead of surrender is because total connection with the subconscious mind can eventually bore you to death! Even though you might want to feel some boredom now and again in order to regain control over your mind's subconscious power, too much boredom and too much subconscious power is no good. Complete boredom unbalances lucid awareness by forbidding a love for life.

In the case of my <u>Earthy</u> lucid dream, the step into boredom turned me around – I simply cooled my overexcitement by focusing on the ground between my feet. As I mentioned, at first my subconscious mind was mesmerized enough to quieten my giddy attitude; then, I got so grounded in boredom that the calmness strained my lucidly aware outlook. I could've kept the dream going by concentrating on something new and interesting; however, I pinched out because I wanted to get my momentary idea about resistive conscious energy written down in my dream diary.

The incredible significance of resisting boredom gets looked at later on. I'll explain why ultimate enlightenment gets strained and drained into total boredom by the flash of ultimate subconscious power coming from a totally submissive attitude. For now, this important idea that conscious and subconscious energy can balance a lucid dream world's deeper mindfulness may be enough of a brain strain; strategies can be planned in the real world since directives can be remembered and acted on while in a lucid dream world.

New ideas occurring in lucid dream worlds can also bring unconventional outlooks back to the real world. Throughout every lucid dream, the individual who attains lucid awareness – only ever one individual at a time – is merged with their deeper dreaming self. Lucid awareness gives rise to conscious belief that the entire dream world has a deeper self – the same "One" self who exists in the real world. After jolting back to my real-world dimension of existence, I can remember and act upon lessons I've learned from lucid dreaming. For example: all seven lucid laws are also about a deeper meaning for conscious survival – in any dimension of reality!

## Transformative Steps

Instead of going two steps backward for every step forward, my upside-down and inside-out, front to back thinking was actually transforming unhealthy attitudes and moods into long-lasting, healthier, and happier ones. I'd really been stepping up and away from shallow mindedness – unawareness of important stuff – by going deeper into my own presence of mind!

After the Earthy lucid dream, I'd always focus on the "ground" the instant I realized I was dreaming. After "grounding" my spirit of overexcitement, I began to bring conscious and subconscious energy back into balance. A balanced mind is all about calming down. Calmer conscious energy makes a person more mindful of subconscious energy. Caring about subconscious energy is an important step that's necessary to keep a lucid dream powered. That's because a caring attitude can control subconscious power.

The way I resist boredom during any dimension of reality has an effect on my mood. The deeper underlying idea behind the Lucid Law of Resistance is all about consciously resisting boredom in ways that feel good for the long-term. The Lucid Law of Resistance is also about resisting the tone of attitude that can antagonize a feel for what's going on. The more antagonized an attitude, the more a person may harmonize with a crappy mood, and then you lose control over your own subconscious power – you can end up suffering through a nightmarish existence during dream worlds and in the real world.

By purposely channelling a caring level of consciousness into any dimension of reality, you can feel the deeper power of a healthier subconscious mood. In other words, a bad mood can unbalance the conscious mind. A good mood can keep the conscious mind going in a healthy direction. Guidance from the Lucid Law of Resistance makes my lucid dreaming last longer because my deceptively unhealthy attitudes transform! Clear as mud, eh? Don't worry, it'll all make sense soon.

Back in my early days of discovery, longer lasting lucid dream worlds always began with me staring at the ground between my feet; then, my ongoing lucid awareness would eventually make me aware of things like the wind rustling leaves on nearby trees, the sounds of birds singing, as well as a sensation of time, and a belief in being somewhere. When I'd finally look up, I'd always feel an appreciation for the pure and natural appearance of my lucid dream world. Conscious focus on a big blue sky filled with puffy white clouds was also mesmerizing for my subconscious mind because I was "cool" with the idea that everything was being created by subconscious energy during a lucidly aware moment!

With a good mood lasting longer, I started moving around more while in a lucid dream world. After calmly realizing that I was in a fantasy of my own creation, an exploration of new dream territory meant there was a lot more subconscious energy to cope with in order to keep the lucid dream going in a direction that felt good for the long-term. Existence in a lucid dream world can become exceedingly painful! I had a steep learning curve ahead of me since it was based on trial and error. After countless gaffes and blunders, I eventually learned – the hard way – how to survive for a very long "time" in a lucid dream world. The good news is that not even the most horrific nightmares could prevent me from eventually jolting back home.

If I wouldn't perform my pinch out move in time, there might be a lot of long-lasting agony. Many of my early attempts to control the lucid dream worlds were terrifyingly violent and bloody! In a real backward stepping way, the scary lucid dream experiences reminded me of the ultra-realistic nightmares I'd suffered through, ever since I was a young child.

Ironically, the Lucid Law of Resistance prevented me from thinking seriously, carefully, or relatively calmly about boredom. That's why there was a long period of time before I accomplished deeper control over my dreaming mind's subconscious energy. As a matter of fact, it was a bunch more years before I began to evolve into a more powerful and mature lucid dreamer; nevertheless, the dream diary recordings of my rough and tumble lucid dream adventures helped (and still help) keep me on a lucid dream – and a real-life – learning curve.

## The Tropical Beach Lucid Dream

Lucid dreams with horrible endings always began innocently enough. For example: the Tropical Beach lucid dream started off fantastically! This dream turned lucid while I ambled along a tropical and exotic stretch of white sand beach. I could hear the open ocean's thunderous waves of rhythmic energy beating against the not so distant resistive outer reef. Except for a pair of flip flops on my feet, I walked bare-naked in the baking heat.

I suddenly wondered: "Where am I?"

Even more important, I asked out loud, "And how did I get here?"

Although everything seemed real as real could be, I wondered if I might be dreaming. Sure enough – I felt that odd sense of dull numbness when I gently pinched my buff backside – lucid dreaming and lucid awareness were confirmed!

Immediately, I stooped forward to focus on the scorching hot sand. The fine loose grains of brownish yellow quartz fragments reminded me of the tiny grains in an hourglass. My overexcited conscious energy receded while I reflected on the idea that these "sands-of-time" were so still. Maybe that was why time seemed to have stopped. Not only that, the strong smell of salty sea air blending with the jungle's earthy aroma made me relish the present moment. I remember feeling myself grinning from ear to ear and laughing out loud with the sheer joy of everything – I was in a lucid dream world!

Eventually, the cry of a seagull woke me from my trancelike state of calmness. I straightened up to face the dazzling realism of calm blue water inside the reef, and all the while the distant surf pounded with a slow, but steady beating on the reef's outer edge. Somehow, I'd managed to lose my flip flops – my only worldly possession. So, I turned back to shore and quickly shuffled up the bright sandy beach in order to keep the bottoms of my feet from burning.

After a long wander under the vibrant, coconut filled palm trees that shaded the beach's higher levels, my big grin was suddenly wiped from my face. My healthy attitude soured when a group of brutishly ugly looking little men poured from the jungle and encircled me. They weren't wearing any clothing either, but these beastlike folks were painted with zigzags of rusty red, muddy brown, and black tinged grime. Along with hearing the thunderous energy of the not so distant ocean waves crashing on the reef, I also felt powerful energy flowing from the stocky natives' waves of anger; every one of them wore a dark expression of cruel hatred!

Three to four feet tall, the stubby brutes each carried a long sharp stick – I was stopped by stinging jabs any time I tried to move or speak. I was sensing the seriousness of the moment. While keeping my hands held up high in order to avoid being "killed" on the spot, a group of meek looking female natives approached from the jungle. Using just their small hands, they quickly dug a deep pit in the stifling sand. The men walked me into the pit, and after the females packed me up to my neck in the oppressive grit, all the natives sauntered off.

The only thing I could do was turn my head from side to side; there was no way for me to perform the pinch out move because my hands were stuck down in the heavy sand. What happened next seemed astonishing: coming into view, I saw dozens of rats scurrying towards me! Although my heart was racing, and I felt a huge adrenaline rush, this terrified subconscious energy was different from the overexcited energy that could jolt me back to the real world. After a lot of shocking pain and agony, this horrific event eventually ended with my blacking out. Without going into the gruesome details of how I felt while being eaten alive by a wave of hungry rats, I'll just say that the experience was really disturbing!

I avoided going insane at the end of the Tropical Beach lucid dream because basic lucid awareness makes me trust that I can't really be killed by a nightmare. Even though no fear of death means there's no freeze response to prevent physical pain, excruciatingly painful episodes occurring in lucid dream worlds usually end with my blacking out (akin to the ending of my Tropical Beach lucid dream). The sudden jolt back to the real world (and my cozy warm bed) always reinforces my belief in the immortality of my deeper dreaming self.

Lucid awareness keeps me linked with my dream world's deeper self, and this link makes me trust that I'll eventually return to another dimension of existence – my real life reality – where a hungry subconscious mind's uncontrolled energy can be just as dangerous!

On a brighter note, my lucid dream worlds were lasting longer and longer, and they were always loaded with adventure. Sometimes a good lucid dream could go on for what seemed like weeks, months or even years when in actuality, after returning home and checking my bedside clock, only a few hours would've passed from when I turned off my bedside lamp! Mornings during long-lasting lucid dream worlds were often blessed with spectacular sunrises, and evenings had the most beautiful sunsets, after which I'd often gaze at stars in the night sky – just like I would in the real world.

In a really long-lasting lucid dream, I'd eventually get into a bed during the lucid dream and fall asleep; this dream sleep would include another pleasant lucid dream world that would keep going for a long period of time, and it in turn would have a sleep period that included even more good lucid dreaming. Deeper and deeper I'd go until ultimately, as though a wave of universal thought reversed itself, I'd start bouncing back from dream sleep to dream sleep, returning to each previous dream world with a jolt. After finally returning home to my real world, I'd often feel as though I'd been gone so long that my real-world reality would feel like the near side – or maybe the "far" side – to another dimension of dreaming!

In my mid thirties, my lucid dreaming really began to evolve. Incredible superhuman stuff like levitating and flying, breathing underwater, changing my own physical form, playing with time, eating and drinking, anything imaginable – even romance with a beautiful woman – all became possible. All this took place because I discovered more basic "lucid laws" for survival in the lucid dream worlds. But, before realizing all seven lucid laws, the authenticity of lucid dreaming created serious challenges – for one thing, I was forced to face my ugliest demons!

For my thirtieth birthday, I went so far as to buy myself a very expensive and very deadly stainless steel replica of a great big old medieval sword that I actually slept with. My plan was to bring an imaginative version of my real-life sword into lucid dream worlds. And I did! Plus, I cut an awful lot of demon's to pieces with it!

I still have the real sword hanging beside my writing desk; it's in a scabbard made by my dear old dad. I spent thousands of hours practice fighting with this sword in my real-world reality, and I remember my dad's hoots of laughter when I told him the real scabbard had to have a clasp. That was because the dream scabbard had to be capable of preventing the dream sword from slipping out if I were flying upside down or diving from great heights while preparing for a "real" fight in a lucid dream world.

I also spent many years practicing a deadly serious martial art – Taekwon-Do – in the real world, thinking that the cunning combat techniques could help me survive longer in a lucid dream world. But, no matter how hard I tried to fight off demons, angry dream brawling turned out to be inharmonious with the way that I wanted to feel. And, dream monsters kept appearing. There was no running or hiding from them – I had to fight the demons else be slain, or even worse – eaten alive! I went through many more gruesome experiences that were similar to the terrifying scene my Tropical Beach lucid dream eventually took me into, all because I couldn't use the pinch and twist technique to escape. I hadn't figured out the rest of the lucid laws, was feeling deeply disturbed about the need for more control over a lucid dream world's subconscious energy.

A lucid dream world feels like the real world; however, the best indicator for differentiating real life from lucid dream life was, and still is, through the gentle pinch test. I often reach a state of mind where I'm not sure whether I'm in the real world or in a lucid dream world unless I perform my pinch test. That's why – in my mid thirties – I considered going for professional help rather than keep suffering my mounting anxiety.

While dawdling over where I could possibly go for help without ending up in a psychiatric ward, a truly amazing lucid dream finally stopped my real-world outlook from filling with what was becoming "out of this world" fear!

## A Soul Saving Lucid Dream

This wild lucid dream began with me standing on a stone ledge near the top of a gentle hill. After staring at the hard rock surface between my feet for so long that time seemed to stand still, I finally calmed down enough to take in the view from my ledge – a beautiful sun-drenched valley was filled with a sea of majestic firs. The sight was stunning, and I felt as though the immediate moment was blooming!

The way the sunlight lit up the valley, the perfect angle of my view, and the wonder I felt from this incredible outlook filled me with awe. My view felt so precious to me because it was energized with so much beauty. Gently sloping and progressing for as far as I could see, the forested valley was alive with songbirds, squirrels leaping about, deer rustling through thick growths of smaller trees and bushes, trickling streams sparkling with reflective light, warm air vibrating with the buzz of insects.

Although I knew I was in a lucid dream world, I felt an extra-special connection with this present moment. All my life, I've loved and treasured the scenic outdoors, yet, more than the view, I suddenly realized that my "present moment" was what felt postcard perfect. I gazed at the beautiful scene for ages. While smiling and nodding my head with tender affection for the heavenly moment, I suddenly understood why my lovely outlook was nourishment for a beautiful mood – I was in a "lucidly loving" presence of mind. Oddly enough, I didn't have a selfish or greedy thought in mind even though I was in a self created lucid dream world; this "lucid love" seemed to just pour out of me without demanding anything in return.

The lucid love that I sent out so freely actually linked the lucid dream world's subconscious energy with the dream world's present moment in a wholesome way. Giving lucid love returns deeper subconscious power – a power to control how the lucid dream world flows!

The "Lucid Law of Love" is the deepest, most upside-down, inside-out, front to back thinking idea coming from all of my lucid dreaming! Not only that, this Lucid Law has become my foundation for guidance in the real world too! It's a challenging concept to understand from a real-world point of view because the Lucid Law of Love isn't limited to conscious energy. The idea behind lucid love is to consciously give love for the present moment – a caring and respectful outlook that can be felt from deep within the subconscious mind.

While in a lucid dream world, I believe that my dream body is subconscious energy because subconscious energy is the fabric for what feels physically real. This way, I can believe that my dream body is a subconscious dream soul. Since my real-world body also feels physically real, I also believe that my real-world body may be defined as a subconscious soul. Conscious energy is different, for instance, lucid love can also take place here in the real world. Lucid love lets me control the kind of subconscious energy that can connect my attitude with deeper happiness. That's why a deeper state of real-world happiness can verify the Lucid Law of Love – easily!

Getting back to that wild <u>Soul Saving</u> lucid dream I was just talking about… when the buzzing insects finally found me, I automatically blew on them in order to shoo them away. My breath made enough wind to clear the bugs, and I noticed nearby tree branches sway in the breeze I'd created.

I thought: "Hmm… I wonder how strong a wind I could make by blowing really hard?" For this reason, I took in a deep breath; then, I blew with all my might. Since I didn't realize I'd tapped into lucid love's control over deeper subconscious power, I was shocked to see trees being uprooted, hear their shattering as they went flying through air filled with erupting black earth; the rock ledge I was on trembled beneath my feet – the whole atmosphere was filled with an insane storm of sound as the entire forest was swept away!

At first, I felt heartbroken because the devastation was complete; my new outlook made me shudder for the loss of "life". The event seemed astounding, but then again, I also felt amazed to wield such power. In the settling silence, I suddenly felt a horrible responsibility for turning this beautiful valley into a dreadful wasteland. I decided to return home, but instead of having to physically pinch out, this time I did it by merely thinking about the pinch out move!

I understood that the entire episode occurred in a lucid dream fantasy and that no real soul was really killed; however, I'd experienced a profound emotion – a loving link with a lucid dream world's present moment – and while writing in my dream diary, I felt the emotion return. Suddenly, I felt a deeper love for my real-world present moment!

My link with lucid love also made me relive the same crushing heartbreak I'd felt at the end of my lucid dream, just before I returned home. And to this day, my memory of that heartbreak is another profound reminder of my growing pains during those years! Even so, I learned that along with the idea of loving the present moment, lucid love's deeper power can transform subconscious energy, enabling me to break free from any tortuous lucid dream event – I only have to think about pinching out from a lucidly loving point of view.

A deeper thinking, more caring, and respectful level of lucid awareness brings me subconscious power to escape from a lucid dream whenever I want. Hallelujah! I could finally stop worrying about the potentially painful and terrifying periods of horror that might occur in my lucid dream worlds. If I couldn't physically perform the pinch out move, all I had to do was think about pinching out from a caring point of view. Sparing myself from having to suffer from so much physical pain and mental agony in my lucid dream worlds – not to mention the despair of a real-world psychiatric ward – made me unearth another powerful and interconnected Lucid Law, the "Lucid law of Tossing Your Burden".

I could "toss the burden" of any antagonized attitude if my outlook was harmonious with lucid love; then, I wouldn't need to escape from a lucid dream world. I could control the way a lucid dream world would flow by loving whatever present moment I was in. All I had to do was toss fear, without upsetting the Lucid Law of Resistance. In other words, I needed to toss my fearful attitudes in ways that wouldn't make the present moment feel boring. Resisting boredom with an attitude free from fear of pain means that I can make a lucid dream world flow in a healthier direction.

Fired up with honest intention to love a lucid dream world's present moment, I can toss burdening conscious and subconscious energy. That's why this Lucid Law of Tossing Your Burden came to light; there's freedom from fear while loving the present moment. The following chapters explain more about the Lucid Law of Love, the Lucid Law of Tossing Your Burden, and the Lucid Law of Resistance while illuminating the other four lucid laws!

CHAPTER TWO

# A STEP FURTHER

Believing that I'd always be able to escape from hurtful events happening in lucid dream fantasies gave me the guts to keep stepping onward – keep exploring a deeper and greater dreaming mind. Healthier dreaming began to take place as I caught more peeks at important pearls of wisdom pouring from long-lasting lucid awareness, long-lasting lucid dream worlds, and longer lasting life!

Everyone and everything within any dream fantasy are expressions of a dreaming mind's imagination. Being a lucidly aware dream soul with the power to return home any time I want, thanks to bringing subconscious energy into balance with lucid love, I've recognized why I also have more than enough imagination to keep a lucid dream going in a good direction.

At the beginning of a lucid dream, I can still feel as though I've hold of a genie's magic lamp; however, a healthier dimension of reality bangs into existence from a deeper thinking rub! During a lucid dream, the real magic is the entire dream world because the fantasy exists during an imaginative present moment.

While in a lucid dream, I'm linked with a deeper self. Although a lucid dream fantasy feels alive, and I want it to live, I believe that such a dimension of existence is a deeper self's presence of mind. Because subconscious energy appears and feels to have a physical presence, I can keep my lucid dream heading in a good direction by loving the dream world's present moment. Once again, the Lucid Law of Love is all about believing in the loveliness of the present moment. What's truly lovely and beautiful may vary depending on a person's preference, but the subconscious mood is similar. A lucidly loving mood doesn't come from a selfish or a greedy attitude; lucid love gets sent out freely because it comes from an actual realization of what I'm imagining to be beautiful.

Understanding the deepest and most powerful Lucid Law of Love means that I can follow a safe path into the deeper power of my subconscious mind. For example: where do you think love comes from? Sensations and emotional moods are states of subconscious energy, yet, I believe that love originates from a conscious attitude. An attitude is conscious, and any attitude that's in harmony with lucid love impresses the subconscious mind with a healthy mood to match.

Loving the present moment enables my deeper self's subconscious mind to create a healthier dream world. Healthier dream world, happier dream life! For me, a healthy dream activity is to fly like Superman. I still love to fly low and slow, above sparkling rivers flowing through lush valleys of dense tropical jungle. Landing for a romantic encounter with a heavenly dream woman is my favourite way to love sharing a beautiful present moment! Floating through such sunny dream worlds, my viewpoint is open to greater subconscious power being controlled by my less resistive conscious mind.

Back in my mid thirties, ideas and understandings pouring from the Lucid Law of Love, Resistance, and Tossing Your Burden enabled me to fill my lucid dream worlds with subconscious energy that was harmonious with loving the lucid dream world's present moment. That's why I came up with the terminology "harmonious joy" in order to describe a healthy subconscious mood. In fact, I had different terminology for lucid love and Lucid Law until recent times, and that's because my lingo has been evolving!

A lucid dream world's mood can also evolve. I can feel healthy subconscious energy that's harmonious with conscious joy when I'm loving the dream world's present moment. Yet, I could still resist boredom in ways that were inharmonious with healthy happiness by feeling a bullying sort of joy – such as feeling superior. Demanding to be obeyed didn't work for long. My bullying type of inharmonious joy came from belief in selfish pride and led to nasty surprises such as the appearance of demonic fiends, phantoms, or monsters who threatened to bring me a world of pain!

I was in my late thirties when one morning, while I added a more readable and detailed account to the previous night's dream diary notes, I finally understood how fellow dream souls could feed fear, anger, and hurt into a lucid dream world – they could enliven my belief in a nightmarish outlook! Since a lucid dream world is an imaginative expression of conscious and subconscious energy, I believed that monstrous demons came from a deeper part of my mind. Since a monster expressed an attitude capable of making a nightmarish outlook feel real for all the dream souls, I'd have to put an end to the bullying sort of joy that was inharmonious with loving my own presence.

I decided to deal with my greatest fears – and monsters – by facing them with a compassionate attitude instead of a sharp sword! A monster could be anything from a crazy giant warrior with fierce fangs and claws, to a ferocious rodent with red-hot eyes, all the way down to a slithering snake with needle-sharp bites. Since a monster was a nasty expression from my own mind, I could toss my fearful attitude by sending compassion toward such a manifestation.

Sure enough, the instant my compassionate point of view stepped forward, everything changed; a threatening and ferocious creature would physically transform into a nicer looking dream soul such as a baby monkey, lion cub, old orang-utan, or an easy going gorilla to name but a few. Telepathically, a transformed monster would ask me to explain who I was, what was happening, and where we were going. Now and then the nicer looking dream soul would hug me or snuggle up and fall asleep. Most often, reduced into submission, the beast would simply gaze at me with the harmlessness of an innocent attitude.

Once again, two steps in a harmoniously joyful direction because of the link with compassion, then another awkward one into my own ignorance. I needed to know more about how to toss burdening energy if I were going to feel truly safe from my demons!

Throughout my late thirties, I began to experience more and more lucid dream life in villages, towns, and cities as they began to trickle into my lucid dream worlds. There were all sorts of dream souls appearing as regular people, and all kinds of interesting relationships took place. The behaviour of regular, everyday folk in my lucid dream worlds seemed healthy. Appearing to be so similar to people in my real world, I kept wondering what was really going on with all the different levels of self-awareness happening all at once in my dreaming mind. The same way most real people seem to be mainly focused on their own individual outlooks, humanlike dream souls were also usually polite, courteous, and sometimes friendly, but mostly focused on their own individual outlooks.

Showing some compassion helped my lucidly loving attitude – and mood – interact with most dream souls in harmoniously joyful ways. Although, some unexpected behaviour from a few of my dream souls led to new pearls of profound insight and wisdom such as: the power of conscious belief, deeper respect for Lucid Law, and more of those down to earth aha moments.

## Reflections

Sometimes, during the course of a lucid dream fantasy, I'll look into a mirror and feel delightfully surprised at seeing a stranger's face looking back! This can occur because taking on a physical form that's different from my real-world body doesn't always happen by choice. Typically, I won't even realize my dream body is different from my real-world body – unless I'm a bird or a fish, or something that's not human.

Usually, I'll have some sort of a human dream body during a lucid dream world. A dream body (dream soul) feels like an elaborate flesh and blood costume – complete with subconscious memories and skills. For example: I've experienced a lot of lucid dreams during which I was an expert guitarist playing incredibly beautiful music at concerts. After returning home, I'd always imagine myself playing these dream songs with real-world musicians, and reproducing masterpieces!

While trying to play guitar in the real world, I've discovered that making good music takes a lot of practice! In order to keep a lucid dream going in a healthy direction, I need to respect the subconscious memories and skills present in my lucidly aware dream soul's "physical" body. A deeper subconscious power – the sort of power enabling me to direct the mood of a lucid dream – arrives when I go along with the way in which the "Lucid Law of Living in the Now" applies to the dream's present moment.

This Lucid Law gets accounted for with more detail and clarity in chapter six; however, for now it's important to understand how and why, similar to real-life souls, dream souls also help maintain the nature of a present moment. The nature of a present moment is all about attitudes, moods, and subconscious skills – such as guitar playing.

To make the most of my lucid dream soul's subconscious skills, I need to keep my attitude in harmony with the Lucid Law of Living in the Now's rule for respecting the presence of deeper subconscious energy. What this boils down to is that I don't resist – in any disrespectful way – the miracle and wonder of a lucid dream world's present moment. Trying to guide the dream world's present moment while disregarding subconscious energy can unbalance my dreaming mind. What I mean is that if I try to take total control with my conscious level of self-awareness, a musical masterpiece won't be happening!

## The Fighter Pilot Lucid Dream

A good example of this "taking control" in a way that ignores guidance from the Lucid Law of Living in the Now took place at the end of the Fighter Pilot lucid dream. At the beginning of this lucid dream, I was strapped into the cockpit of a super sleek jetfighter. Through the front of the cockpit canopy, I could see that my warplane was set on the deck of an aircraft carrier!

Subconsciously, I already knew that my heavily armed fighter was hooked up to a high tech, high pressure steam catapult, and that I was preparing for a launch. I remember watching my fingers flicking switches and pressing buttons automatically, without my having to think; the cockpit was filled with complex looking dials and screens, and a deep sounding macho voice was speaking a specialized military lingo on the headset inside of my flight helmet.

I felt calm, as though on autopilot, no pun intended. Indeed, lucid awareness linked this present moment with my dream world's deeper self, and I marvelled at my new outlook. The experience was a lot like watching a movie, except I was actually in this one. Then again, I was thinking that flying a warplane into battle might disrespect the Lucid Law of Love since a war's mood was mostly fearful, angry, and hurtful. I still had to learn that a deeper level of respect for the present moment gives healthy direction for subconscious energy. This Lucid Law of Living in the Now is also about guiding subconscious energy in a healthy direction.

When a ground crew guy performed a snappy salute, my free hand automatically returned the compliment; my other hand gripped a swivelling lever with lots of buttons near my thumb – the control stick. Then slam! I felt a terrific force stuff me into the back of my seat. I watched the ship's bow come speeding toward me while a blur of colour flashed by in my peripheral.

After the jetfighter cleared the deck, I took conscious control over the control stick. Instead of letting the lucid dream character's subconscious mind – without my thinking about it – fly the fighter, I'd taken control in a disrespectful manner because I'd no idea how to fly a jetfighter. That's why there could be no harmony between me and control over this plane of existence!

As though suddenly jamming on a car's brake, I stomped down on a foot pedal: one pedal went down while another came up. After the jet turned sharply, I yanked back on the control stick; the aircraft was responding to my every command. In sickeningly slow motion, an upside-down, dark blue sea seemed to be spinning toward me... I was going to crash! I instantly wished to return home and automatically "ejected" out of the lucid dream world with that familiar jolt. I escaped just as the jetfighter pan-caked (upside-down) into the ocean.

Linking with guiding power from the Lucid Law of Living in the Now allows subconscious skills within my lucidly aware dream soul to help keep the lucid dream "alive". There's a depth of trust involved with how much control to take. Just like every conscious real-world soul, a conscious dream soul performs unthinking subconscious skills automatically. Things like walking and running, riding a bicycle or a horse, playing a musical instrument, or even flying a plane need to be treated with respect. Taking control often comes down to guiding the present moment in a healthy direction. Trying to take over and micromanage the "physical" dream world doesn't work!

Then again, sometimes I don't inhabit a dream body at all. But, as long as I observe the Lucid Law of Living in the Now, and share the present moment in a caring and respectful way – I'm guiding my subconscious mind in a healthy direction. That's because my subconscious mind powers every dream soul, enabling a deeper subconscious mood to channel harmoniously joyful viewpoints.

A happy movie usually has healthy moods in mind for the audience, and the actors' attitudes (imaginative states of conscious energy that the audience loves to gobble up) feed the audience these moods. Similarly, I can keep my lucid awareness and lucid dream world happy by feeding the lucid dream world healthy attitudes. Even without a dream body, I'm able to feed a stream of lucidly loving energy into my dream world's present moment, empowering the dream characters with good moods that I can feel.

Knowledge and understanding gained from the many different moods felt during lucid dream worlds brings me greater insight about deeper reasons for the moods in these new planes of existence. A clear case of such greater insight happened during the course of an especially special erotic lucid dream!

## An Especially Special Erotic Lucid Dream

During an Especially Special Erotic lucid dream, even the prettiest women were more than just attracted to me – they were down right head over heels smitten at first sight! As I walked along a busy city sidewalk, I felt a bit taken aback because so many beautiful women kept glancing my way; I hadn't yet realized that I'd taken on a new physical form.

I quickly turned off the sidewalk, strode up a long paved driveway with high and neatly trimmed cedar hedges on either side, and found myself walking into a huge gothic mansion – a long-standing place made from what looked to be thick slabs of silvery speckled granite. There were massive wooden staircases, some curving and spiralling up and up into darker and ever deepening passageways. Best of all, there was a warm, festive, and party like atmosphere about the place. All sorts of men and women were lounging around, and the women were being a lot more than just friendly!

More to the point... later on in this lucid dream, I was on the run! An aggressive and nightmarishly nasty woman was chasing after me when I happened to glance at my reflection in a huge hallway mirror. I felt delightful surprise because a strikingly handsome man was looking back! I stopped and stared. This dream soul was different from my real-world soul: clean shaven, square jawed and with high cheekbones, large and widely spaced cobalt blue eyes, thick wavy black hair, and a stunningly muscular naked body, the reason why I was getting an overwhelming amount of attention from the ladies wasn't hard to figure out!

Lucid awareness made me understand that everyone and everything were expressions from my own dreaming mind. That's why I played along with the mind game in a harmoniously respectful manner. By going along with guidance from the Lucid Law of Living in the Now, I discovered how another's attitude can have an enormous influence on my individual mood.

In my Especially Special Erotic lucid dream, I felt passionate about romantic connections with attractive female dream souls; our flesh and blood "costumes" were perceived as being beautiful, and our individual moods were alive with exquisite pleasure! The reason why a conscious belief in lust can have such a powerful influence on a body's mood is because as I explained earlier, a person's subconscious mind can feel uplifting subconscious energy if their conscious mind is interpreting the moment as being beautiful. Beauty appears in the eye of the beholder because beauty comes from the beholder's belief.

A belief impresses the subconscious mind, and the subconscious responds with a mood that has an effect on the conscious mind. Yet, this Especially Special Erotic lucid dream – in which so many women seemed to believe that they were in love with my dream soul – revealed a profound insight about the concept of an even deeper dimension of conscious energy relative to real-life reality, let alone dream reality!

As I gazed into the huge hallway mirror and saw such a handsome man, I suddenly understood why a belief in physical beauty can generate more than just lustful love. A deep pleasure comes from conscious belief in what looks good, what feels cute and cuddly, along with what smells, tastes, or sounds attractive. Conscious belief can also set the stage for subtle, dangerous, and inevitable traps. Case in point: by believing in loveliness, most people also accept a shadow side – ugliness – as being real.

My reflection gave me a deeper reason to pause and consider feeling some compassion for the unattractive dream soul that I was fleeing from. Stopping to gaze at my unfamiliar, yet, extraordinarily handsome reflection, I experienced one of those down-to-earth "aha" moments! My reflection brought me an answer for the appearance of all my ugly demons: individual levels of consciousness can become selfishly sinister if their soul is channelling unhealthy truth behind conscious belief! Without any associated feelings of deeper love or real respect for the present moment, the unattractive dream soul appeared to be in an ugly mood, and came after me like a demon! That's why I finally escaped from her by purposely pinching out – I wanted to record my aha moment in my dream diary!

A lucidly loving feel for the moment I'm experiencing during any dimension of reality arrives with my giving respect for whomever or whatever I'm imagining to be beautiful. Lucid love is also about giving respect and showing compassion for a present moment that I'm imagining to be ugly.

At this stage in my explanation about how to get deeper subconscious power from understanding more about lucid love, there's an idea that a subconscious mood connects the conscious mind with emotional feelings. Being aware of my mood helps me glimpse a clearer picture of what's really going on in my own subconscious mind because consciousness enables me to respect powerful subconscious emotions.

Every dream fantasy is about a lot more than just seeing, hearing, smelling, tasting, and touching what I make-believe to be real because a dream is also about making moods feel real. Being aware of my present real-life mood helps me realize an equivalent meaning behind what's really going on with attitudes here in the real world. Conscious belief can bring powerful emotions to life!

Experiencing loveliness and ugliness during dream worlds happens all the time, and these same experiences also take place in the real world. After that <u>Especially Special Erotic</u> lucid dream took place, I marvelled at how every real person could easily feel lucid love heal an unhealthy and unhappy outlook. Lucid love's deeper power is subconscious because the subconscious mind makes belief feel real. Subconscious power is vital for shaping good and bad outlooks, good and bad moods, good times and bad times happening in dream worlds and in the real world. Going deeper into the idea that a subconscious mind is physical reality while a conscious mind is the "time of your life" steps us straight into the next Lucid Law, which arrives right off the bat in the next section!

## The Recurring Nightmares

During dreams and in the real world, your own subconscious mind makes your beliefs feel real. That's why another important Lucid Law is the "Lucid Law of Belief".

The Lucid Law of Belief is all about how an individual level of consciousness feels real. This Lucid Law is also concerned with why a belief has an effect on a viewpoint. More specifically, certain "actual" events having occurred in dream worlds may feel real for your subconscious memory. Subconscious memory is all the stuff you've forgotten about, but remains buried deep in your mind – in a place that's normally disconnected from conscious energy.

Some folks don't remember anything about their dream worlds, yet, scientific studies show that REM (rapid eye movement – under closed eyelids) during sleep periods correlates with dreaming. Not only that, by constantly waking a person from their REM sleep, and preventing their dreams from happening, after one week the person begins to suffer from psychotic behaviour; then, after being allowed to dream again, the person's sanity returns.

The instant you wake up, instead of immediately focusing on what time it is, or on your upcoming day, you're capable of thinking about the previous night's dream worlds. Writing about dreams in a dream diary also helps reconnect the conscious mind with subconscious memory from REM sleep, making the recollection feel as though the events were real. Your subconscious mind remembers a perception of any good times, bad times, or boring times, and these perceptions then loop back to verify (or modify) your belief about what was really happening.

Whether a conscious belief originates in the real world or in a dream world, the mood you were in happens to be a significant part of your belief system. For example: if you were feeling healthy while dreaming, your recollection of the dream would be from a different point of view than if you were feeling sick, scared, or miserable.

Using your senses to get information about the surrounding environment or situation helps you perceive where you are and what's going on. Discovering how to feel good about what's going on wherever you are – right now – can begin by focusing clearly and intuitively on the spirit of your present attitude. Recognizing the nature of your attitude helps bring a deeper understanding about the Lucid Law of Belief because you'll become more aware of how your present attitude acts upon your subconscious mood, sometimes causing your mood to change.

I've discovered a multitude of parallels to link the idea that moods and memory happening in the real world are comparable with moods and memory happening during dream worlds. Straight to the point, these parallels are made evident in the way a person's memory of a dream world can act upon their real-world subconscious mood, and cause it to change!

Most people believe that their brain creates their awareness of what's going on. I used to think that my brain created my self-awareness for the reason that my brain is separate and individual. That's why I believed that my mind was also separate and individual. Yet, my lucid dream worlds have made me recognize why I had it backwards. That's because dream souls can channel a universal presence of mind, and make it feel individual!

A lucidly aware dream soul's brain doesn't create that soul's self-awareness, their soul (which includes a brain) channels a subconscious present moment into a conscious present moment. While in a lucid dream world, I believe that my subconscious mind is the dream world's space-time continuum because along with guidance coming from the Lucid Law of Belief's really important ideas and understandings, I've realized how and why there's a universally aware subconscious mind at work during all dream worlds!

Next, sharing a very special set of recurring nightmares I went through illustrates this concept of seemingly individual levels of consciousness actually being the same universal self-awareness. Even though they really were rough and tumble, I'll always cherish those five dream experiences which clearly demonstrate how and why an individual body and soul (and brain) can channel a conscious belief in having a separate personality. This way, a conscious belief in being a separate soul feels real. Lucid dreaming reveals why there's a lot more to consciousness than just belief in being an individual!

My wake-up call began a little later in life (late thirties) after a conclusive nightmare streamed from four recurring ones, none of which could ever be ignored, forgotten, or denied. That's because I wrote down the experiences in my dream diary! Ironically, these backward flowing nightmares got me stepping onward, toward a new belief in the deeper power of everyone's subconscious mind.

Four nights in a row, I dreamt that I was a serf who lived in the medieval era. Each recurring dream began in an ancient and peaceful village where we villagers were suddenly attacked by dozens of knights on horseback! After setting fire to the village, armoured nobles raised their giant sized medieval swords to slash at panic stricken peasants. As our close knit shacks burned, I remained in the middle of the settlement square – frozen with fear. The heavy stench of crackling smoke blackened the village in more ways than one as this was a dark ending to an old way of life. People screamed and animals freaked out – even the ground I stood upon trembled beneath the knights' charging horses!

Night after night, these non-lucid dream worlds seemed like a genuine real-life reality for me. Linked with the serf's soul, I felt terrified throughout the first three nightmares – my heart raced and throat constricted: the serf couldn't move, could hardly even breathe, let alone cry out for help. There was so much fearful conscious and subconscious energy streaming within his paralyzed dream body that I could barely believe what was happening. I wanted to escape, but my arms and legs felt heavy as lead.

Without the possibility for fight or flight, a belief in certain death can cause a third physical reaction to take place – freeze! Same as freezing you into place in the real world, an emotional fear of death can also cause a dream soul's body to "freeze" into place!

After returning home (and waking up) from each of the first three nightmares, the experiences were recorded in my dream diary. While reading over the notes that I wrote so long ago, a memory of the age-old village returns without difficulty. The first three of the recurring nightmares were filled with an unhealthy fear of death because I never achieved lucid awareness.

All four of the nightmares (plus the fifth and concluding one) ended with my sudden jolt back to my real-world bedroom. After rousing from each of the first three, I wrote about immense surprise and huge relief for having escaped the horror. Instant release from such fear felt fantastic.

Although I didn't enter into lucid awareness during any of the first three recurring nightmares, the experiences still seemed incredible! Those nightmares were trying to tell me something important; however, their real meaning remained a mystery until the fourth night… the fourth nightmare started off the same as the first three except for one major difference: while the village was under attack, I felt a staggering sensation of compassion. My fearful perception of what was going on around me began to transform as a respect for the villagers and our rustic way of life welled up within my heart. Next, my fear gave way to an overwhelming belief that a devastating injustice was taking place! I began to breathe deeper and thought, "How can I stop these monsters on horseback from destroying the community?"

All at once, my old mood shattered, and since I still believed there was no way to escape, a mood of hot anger erupted. With new subconscious energy firing up from my new belief, my first furious move was to grab a familiar garden hoe that was on the ground beside me; I would fight to prevent this terrible event from continuing.

Raging, my voice howled and roared over the horrendous injustice taking place! Immediately, a huge black horse wearing an armour breastplate loomed out of the smoke. Feeling a surge of adrenaline, I thrust my gardening tool upward, aiming for the steely knight who rode high upon the enormous animal.

The flash of a silver blade caught my attention, but it took me a sec before I realized that the knight's sword had just nicked me in the neck. Hot blood was spurting out of my dream body! The knight returned a backhanded stroke of his sword, and he began to hack me down.

This powerful knight appeared magnificent in a sinister sort of way since he wore a great shiny metal helmet with a red dragon painted above the eye slit. I looked through the slit and straight into his blazing blue eyes. After our awareness of one another seemed to lock together, I knew that the brutal blows from his sword would continue cutting me to pieces! I grasped the horror of it all while falling to my knees; then, I felt my body melting into the ground.

Not knowing that I was also at home, in bed, and asleep, my mind had me responding to a world that I believed was real. An angry level of self-awareness was fully engaged with the action of the moment. My individual mood sank deeper into the realism of the dream's present moment because I consciously believed that I was in an objective world – a world based on facts that existed independently of my own mind.

There was the objective truth that deadly sword strikes continued to bite me; then, the muscle tension in the remains of my dream body released entirely, and I felt kind of good. Floating up and out of my corpse, I felt free from all my anger, fear, and hurt since I hadn't died! I was still conscious, and a belief that I was still alive changed my entire outlook. My consciousness drifted higher and higher. Incredibly, I could feel emotions from everybody beneath. While sensing each "living" dream soul's subconscious energy, my consciousness expanded beyond belief! As the slaughter raged, the moment felt profound as well as passionate. Oddly enough, I sensed an immense burst of anguish from the knight who had just slain my serf's soul.

A corner of my conscious mind struck upon the idea that a deeper presence was channelling a nasty present moment. Floating upward and outward, while reaching inward, a clearer perception of self-definition began to emerge. Although I was still feeling intense energy flowing within all of the individual dream souls, I felt calm as well as thankful for my greater outlook. My sensing each individual soul's subconscious energy was helping to keep my serf's consciousness alive!

With a sudden snap, my serf's expanding level of self-awareness turned lucid. Lucid awareness brought me an immediate realization that the whole event was a dream! Miraculously, I understood why I was every one of those living dream souls. Concurrently, each dream soul was an individual expression of the same dreaming mind. Arriving from another dimension of reality, my dreaming mind's subconscious energy was the fabric for: all the individual dream souls, the village, sky, fields, forest, and everything else feeling physically real. I also realized that the entire dream world's present moment was my dreaming mind's deeper self-awareness.

As though energized by a lightning bolt, my expanding and lucidly aware point of view hit upon a wondrous level of enlightenment – everything seemed so simple and straightforward because I'd grasped a more magnificent meaning behind all of my dream worlds! Since my serf's dream body was gone, my new outlook was universal: a deeper level of self-awareness was flowing in a stream of infinite subconscious power. Although everything happened really fast, I remember realizing that this outlook was so quick and powerful because without a belief in embodiment, I no longer felt a resistance to anything!

After returning home with a jolt, I sat up, switched on the bedside light, and in a flash my dream diary was in my hands. I wrote and wrote, and wrote. Alas, getting my enlightened outlook down on paper wasn't practical at that time – seven books and decades of serious consideration would be required!

Although I believed that something miraculous had happened to me during that fourth recurring nightmare, this was only the beginning of a pivotal awakening into a new belief in deeper self-definition. That's because I was starting to perceive the incredible power within my dreaming mind. Before this night was through, plenty more would be written because another remarkable dream, also briefly lucid near the end, took place after I fell back to sleep.

## The Clincher Lucid Dream

The <u>Clincher</u> lucid dream had me dressed in armour. This dream was the clincher for all those recurring medieval nightmares. My <u>Clincher</u> lucid dream began with my dream soul holding a gigantic medieval sword in one gauntleted hand – sharp tip pointed high. Riding a huge galloping horse, reins were held in my other hand as I reigned supreme from a belief in being above all others in power, authority, rank, status, skill, and quality of consciousness. That's because as I said, I didn't link with lucid awareness until near the end of this final medieval dream.

Along with me, a brotherhood of knights rode upon big battle scarred warhorses. We would enforce our rule of the land upon everything in our path! Filled with a belief in my moral superiority, and feeling mighty proud about it, I rode out front.

Bright and early during this cool morning, the smell of leather was strong, and the sound of rattling equipment complimented the rhythmic feel of my mighty horse's gallop. Through the eye slit in my helmet, I could see an onrushing dirt path. The idea that I was a genuine knight in shining armour seemed natural and normal. Additionally, my dash along this dirt passageway felt familiar. Subconsciously, I knew that there was an upcoming bend in the path and that I'd have to rein in my steed.

Sure enough, my horse slowed his pace and we made the turn. Next, there came a shallow but fast flowing river. Splashing onward, I could hear the following knights' lively horses prancing through the frigid torrent. Although I felt proud of my role as leader, I also felt a deeper and more frigid chill than that of the river. Flowing deep down in the heart of my individual dream soul, I'd a feeling that this was going to be an exceptionally brutal mission.

After crossing the river, we descended into a lushly forested valley of vibrant green, and I worried about falling into a trap: serious shadows were potential hiding places for resentful peasants who could be armed with stolen bows and arrows. I gripped my gigantic medieval sword more tightly; the sword felt light as a feather and remained at the ready. With the sharp tip pointed straight up, a quick centre block movement of this over-size broadsword would stop any heavy arrow fired at my helmet's eye slit – a vulnerable spot in my armour.

A sensation of imminent danger soared as the sleepy village, a rebellious place where taxes had been left unpaid, appeared directly before us. Luckily, surprise was still on our side! We were there to punish the peasants for not paying community taxes. An effective fear of further arrest, devastation, and death would keep law, order, and taxes flowing in similar villages throughout the land.

I waggled my sword – an attack signal – before belting out a mighty howl that made my helmet ring. Obediently, all of the knights attacked the village! The dawn sky soon grew dark with raunchy smelling smoke; then, the villagers' small huts began to burst into huge balls of fiery red flames.

Shortly after the eruption of panicked and screaming medieval farm workers, I came upon a feisty and mean-tempered looking serf. Barefoot and dressed in dirty old pants and shirt, he stood before me, jabbing upward with a ridiculous garden tool. I presumed this worthless peasant must be part of the tax rebellion; instead of arrest, I'd strike him down for his violent insolence.

The tip of my sword nicked the lowly serf's neck, and I saw – with a mounting feeling of foreboding – his blood spurting out. My powerful arm seemed to have a will of its own, kept slashing the huge broadsword at the stunned looking fellow. Just before he fell, I caught him staring straight into my eyes. Suddenly, I recognized him – he was me!

Bewildered and dumbfounded, I recognized another version of myself: his body was tall and slim just like mine, his long wavy hair was auburn, his beard crimson and clipped short, nose modest, plus his big blue eyes were also exactly like mine. I felt an overwhelming sensation of confusion mix with my dark surprise, and then this intense feeling of respect for the man tangled with a belief in the righteousness of my sword arm.

Some compassion finally arrived, and I wanted to stop the butchery. Mystified with my lack of control, I couldn't understand why my arm wouldn't stop swinging the bloodied sword. As the fellow fell to the ground, a cry of agony wailed within my helmet! Tears burst down my face as I cried out: "What the hell is going on?!?"

Abrupt lucid awareness suddenly made me realize that I was dreaming. I could finally stop striking and hacking. I actually let go of the colossal sword, watched it fall to the earth while at the same time, I felt awestruck at how incredibly real everything seemed. Screams and smoky smells coming from the slaughter faded into the background as I focused on the chopped mess down below.

With a lucid level of self-awareness in place, I zoomed in on a deeper meaning to this lucid dream. There was no longer any mystery as to why my arm kept swinging that sword: part of me didn't want to merge with my deeper dreaming self, didn't want to recognize that a dreaming self from another dimension of existence was every dream soul's deeper self. The egotistical knight in shining armour was subconsciously trying to cut the possibility of a link with lucid awareness because his level of self-awareness wanted to believe in supremacy and a heightened impression of self-importance.

Lucid awareness transformed the knight's egotistical outlook. Not only that, I realized how a shielded version of the same "One" dreamer's self-awareness could make a conscious dream soul believe in being individual. I understood that such knowledge could also answer many age-old questions about the nature of all dimensions of existence because I realized how all the seemingly separate dream souls were the same deeper self! Then there came a brisk jolt back to my real world.

Sitting bolt upright in bed, I switched the light on for the second time that night. Another rare occasion is turning the light on after returning from a dream world because just jotting down a few notes in the dark is usually enough of an effort. But this was another of those extraordinary lucid dream fantasies, even though it was only briefly lucid at the end.

With eyes wide open, a whole new concept dawned on me: my deeper thinking presence of mind presented a "whole" new way to view my real world! While writing about the deeper level of lucid awareness I'd just experienced at the end of my <u>Clincher</u> lucid dream, I stepped into a deeper, real-life presence of mind. I even gave a name to my new presence of mind – "Front To Back Thinking".

My real-life, Front To Back Thinking (FTBT) mindset comprehended a clearer concept of dream world conscious energy because all seemingly separate levels of self-awareness are the same deeper self. This fifth and conclusive medieval dream showed me that a dream soul channels a level of the dreamer's self-awareness!

Moods and memory help create a perception of individual self-definition – a belief in being individual further impacts moods and memories. But, moods and memories can change due to belief, and vice-versa – belief can change due to moods and memories! As long as who you think you are is defined by a belief that you're an individual level of consciousness, your subconscious memory of deeper self-awareness can remain shielded. This way, you may consciously believe that your individual level of self-awareness is your only self.

A human soul's conscious belief in exaggerated self-importance, often accompanied by excessive aggressiveness, actually compensates for an accompanying fear of death. Bullies – both male and female – who believe in being mighty, righteous, and proud enforcers of their own selfish viewpoints can display an unhealthy truth behind a belief in supremacy – fear of their own death. What's more, a superiority-complex can lack respect and empathy for those seen as inferior.

Awareness of nightmarish existence can also arrive by consciously believing in being inferior. Belief that I was an inferior serf made my fear of being killed by a superior knight feel so intense that my serf's subconscious soul froze from the fearful feedback! But, lucid awareness revealed how and why – within a dream world – each and every level of self-awareness is actually equal instead of being superior or inferior. That's because every dream soul (unless lucid) channels a shielded level of another self – the deeper dreaming self.

Tuning into this concept of every dream soul's unique level of self-awareness actually being a multidimensional dreaming self made me understand why, no matter what the status, the significance of each dream soul's self-awareness is equal. This new understanding also brought to light how all the fear, anger, and hurt that I'd felt throughout those medieval nightmares really resulted from my conscious belief in an ugly present moment being real!

Causing disagreement and hostility capable of splitting any group's unity, a conscious belief in a different depth of self-awareness being either superior or inferior makes a selfish attitude feel greedy for superiority. Every dream soul has a certain depth of self-awareness, yet, unless lucidly aware, each soul is shielded from their deeper self – the dreamer. This way, there's serious competition to stay alive! Plus, most victors in any game of survival tend to believe that they're extraordinarily special, while "losers" are thought to be less significant.

The fourth and fifth medieval dreams expanded my viewpoint because I realized that the same dreamer "lives" a dream world through all of the dream souls – all at the same time! This new perception changed my belief in what self-definition is all about as I was suddenly conscious of a lot more than how a multidimensional mind can create a dream world. That's because I understood why – during a dream world – no "One" can be second-rate.

Since everyone's self-awareness – during a dream world – streams within the same dreaming mind, the dream souls are equal in the "realness" of their self-awareness. An individual dream soul isn't superior or inferior in self-awareness because every "One" is the same self. Each dream soul appears to have their own shielded and guarded mindset – a veiled version of their deeper dreaming mind; however, most dream souls are shallow minded due to an ignorance of who they really are!

The amplified feeling of unity that both the serf and knight eventually experienced when their consciousness became lucid made me understand something profoundly universal, but also very individual. During any dream world, a universally aware subconscious mind energizes and feels the dream world while simultaneously, the same presence of mind "lives" the creation from individual points of view. Happening all at the same time, veiled and guarded levels of self-awareness can feel real!

My deeper, real-life FTBT (Front To Back Thinking) made me realize that the same thing could be happening in the real world! That's because

FTBT makes me look at, question, test, and reflect upon there being a deeper self here in the real world too. A deeper thinking mindset also suggests that there's an ignorance of who we really are in the real world!

So, who are we really? Realizing that a limited perception of who you really are makes your dream reality feel perfectly real can help you understand why a limited perception of who you really are also makes your real world feel perfectly real!

Purposely transforming a belief in being no more than an individual level of self-awareness – one who is either superior or inferior to everyone else in the real world – helps step you onward… toward a deeper and increasingly more powerful belief in the equality of all self-awareness. All the separate levels of a real-life philosophical puzzle can fit together to create a clearer perception of who we all really are – the same "One" deeper self!

CHAPTER THREE

# DREAM REVIEWS AND REVELATIONS

The colourful whirling and twirling planet Earth is truly miraculous. Beyond everything happening on such a beautifully blue planet, we're orbiting a big bright sun, and this dazzling sun spirals within a star studded galaxy. Not only that, the sun helps to light a path throughout an expanding cosmos where a wondrous dimension of existence is real-life reality! What's more, along with all the commotion going on in the universe, our planet Earth is alive with the brilliance – and dizziness – of conscious and subconscious energy!

While pondering upon the vastness of the universe, let alone the depth of eternity, how can you come up with a meaningful and self-empowering view on the true meaning of life? Say what? Why in the world would you want to think about all that true meaning of life stuff?

One whopper of a reason for catching a glimpse at what's really going on with conscious and subconscious energy is that you get to experience the most massive aha moment imaginable! By discovering a deeper point for the existence of conscious and subconscious energy, you also get to play with deeper subconscious power – thanks to an astounding leap in enlightenment!

Even though your individual level of real-world self-awareness may have been shocked by heartbreak, injustice, ugliness, or a fear of death, you can still catch more than just a fleeting glimpse of deeper self-awareness. That's because the real meaning of dreaming matches the real meaning of life. Bringing conscious and subconscious energy into balance makes a healthy presence of mind feel real; a lucidly aware point of view can explain the reason why.

With regards to real-world self-awareness, a balanced presence of mind helps you transcend your own emotional pain in order to ask some meaningful questions such as: "What exactly is self-awareness anyway? Why am I here? Where has everything come from?" These sorts of questions – along with other important personal issues – may be resolved by stepping your individual level of self-awareness onward, into deeper reasoning discovered through deeper thinking lucid awareness. For example: in place of irrational, vague, or uncertain hope of there being a point to your life, understanding why we're all here feels far, far more comforting!

While in a dream world, you and the other conscious dream characters that you interact with usually have no concept of a multidimensional subconscious mind. You may feel as though everything is perfectly real during a dream world because unless you're lucid, you won't recognize that you're in a dream – it's only after waking up that you can realize you were dreaming.

Even though at times things may seem weird, unfamiliar, or disturbing, people usually remember a dream world from only one point of view, as if being a real-life individual who's living a real dimension of reality. This way, imaginary dream souls, dream scenes, and dream events appear to be a genuine dimension of existence while the dream is happening. Immediately after waking up, you may remember a dream occurrence for a short period before dismissing the significance of such an event – since it was a figment of imagination.

On the other hand, a lucid dream feels different. As I explained in chapter one, the lucidly aware dream character can control their dream world's subconscious energy – the dreamer's subconscious mind. For me, keeping my lucid dream world going in a healthy direction comes about by reflecting on the seven lucid laws (one at a time) while I'm dreaming. This way, my dream world gets impressed by my conscious intention to love the lucid dream world's present moment, which includes loving the idea that I can toss any fearful, angry, and hurtful resistance to having a good time!

Five of these lucid laws have been touched upon so far: the Lucid Law of Resistance, Love, Tossing Your Burden, Living in the Now, and Belief. Going along with the healthy truth behind even one Lucid Law prevents suffering from the truth behind any of the others. That's because lucid love has a positive effect on subconscious energy.

## The Albatross Lucid Dream

The <u>Albatross</u> lucid dream brings insight into the significance of subconscious energy. Taking place in my late thirties, this lucid dream began in fresh sunshine, above a clean and bright blue sea, and I felt exhilarated to be flying! My lucid awareness was energized with love and respect for the dream world's present moment – I knew I was a bird, a big one too!

Everything about being this big bird felt normal and familiar since my direction of thought in the dream world was in harmony with guidance developed from the Lucid Law of Living in the Now. That's why, by allowing my dream soul's subconscious mind to flex feathered wings over and over again, I seemed to swim through the warm summer sky. As well, my body felt healthy and strong; then, there came my delightful surprise at seeing a sailing ship (with three tall masts) on the horizon in front of me!

By loving the bird's present moment of existence, I went along with the Lucid Law of Living in the Now and flowed with lucid love's incredible subconscious power to control the lucid dream world. In addition, my idea to board the sailing ship directed my immediate course. With an amazed spirit of wonder, my mood was filled with an intense pleasure as I glided down, down towards the gilt-edged stern of the old square-rigger.

I floated on a luxurious tail wind, through warm and astonishingly clear air. My approach from behind the vessel allowed me to classify her as an eighteenth century era frigate. Levelling out a few meters above an expansive sea of subconscious energy, I noticed that the ship had a lengthy row of closed gun-port lids along her sunlit side, the side that I intended to pass. These large-scale, closed lids hinted at dozens of heavy cannons on board.

The same gentle breeze carrying me also waved an old-fashioned British flag above the frigate's stern where the name <u>UNICORN</u> stood out in bright, bold, gold lettering. At the same time, the warm wind filled inaudible clouds of great billowed sails that pressed the ship onward. Here was the spirit of adventure – a commanding sight to behold!

Owing to my keen enthusiasm about square-rigged sailing ships and the amazing people that made them sail, this was a golden opportunity to experience a new adventure! By managing the way the dream unfolded, I could become an officer on the quarterdeck, maybe even the captain of the ship!

Closer and closer to the ship I flew, until I heard sea water slapping against her wood hull. While she shouldered her way through a wave, there was the savage squeal of block and tackle as burly sailors worked to adjust intimate webs of taut rigging.

I savoured the moment in order to manage my excitement. A change in physical form meant that my lucid awareness would slip from the bird's point of view and land on the ship's quarterdeck where I would get a whole new outlook. But, while briefly focusing down on the sparkling water so as to maintain my lucid awareness, I lacked the calm expectation necessary to be certain of joining the ship's company. I felt that something wasn't quite right – everything seemed so real. I needed to keep focusing on loving to share the present moment in order to make my transformation happen. But, I was feeling uncertain about my intention to become an officer, preferably the sailor in command. An underlying unhealthy truth was all about greed for superiority.

Any conscious uncertainty signals that I'm in violation of my own onboard guidance coming from Lucid Law. Uncertainty or lack of intention can keep me stuck in doubt. Uncertainty, indecision, and doubt serve to mark the beginning of the end for controlling my direction during a lucid dream world, whereas confidence empowers a "profound feel for intention". A profound feel for intention amounts to that feeling of certainty coming from trusting that you're going in the right direction!

In the case of the <u>Albatross</u> lucid dream, once I was aboard the Unicorn, a new path would be set; however, I wasn't ready to give up my bird's eye point of view just yet. My involvement with lucid dreaming was still on a steep learning curve, and I loved this view. While flying past the starboard side of the ship, I saw a few of the seagoing officers pointing toward me and heard one cry out, "Albatross ho!"

A sharp banking turn had me crossing her bow, and I was suddenly assaulted by what I perceived to be a disgusting stench! The reek of several hundred filthy men was so surprisingly disagreeable that my wavering idea to get onboard was suddenly belayed. I automatically focused on the pinch out move in order to jolt back home.

Fortunately for me, my belief in a raw smell being too ugly to tolerate probably saved me from a lucid nightmare. The next morning, after checking out my dream diary, a deeper focus on the <u>Albatross</u> lucid dream experience made me wonder if interpreting a smell as being shockingly horrible could be due to an unhealthy truth behind a belief? There was an unhealthy truth about the real Albatross around my neck because the deeper truth that a warship fight for belief in superior outlooks was what really stunk! Firepower for defence is one thing, for selfish greed it's another shot in the wrong direction!

Once again, a lucid dream helped me step out of an unhealthy real-life outlook. A healthier outlook arrives when, instead of intending to fight for love, I intend on giving love with no strings attached.

## **Lucid Awareness**

A total merge with a deeper presence of mind channels lucid awareness, and the dream turns into a lucid one. Although existence during a lucid dream world feels real, lucid awareness makes me believe that such realism resonates by subconscious design. While in a lucid dream world, a self-aware, yet, individualistic expression of imaginative energy – usually me in an imaginary replica of my real-world body – merges with a deeper level of self-awareness than that of fellow dream characters.

While lucidly aware, I believe that I'm much more than just a dream soul. Enlightenment occurs because having lucid awareness compels me to align and completely merge with every soul's deeper self, the "One" who sleeps safely in another dimension relative to the dream world.

As a consequence of aligning and merging with my dream world's deeper self, control over subconscious energy brings me the ability to channel my desires and needs into existence. If I want to fly for example, since I'm loving the dream world's present moment, I can control the dream world's gravitational energy, enable my humanoid dream soul to float off the ground and command instant travel through the air. Or, if I need to eat, go to the toilet, or even go to bed and sleep, I can. It's possible for me to do anything imaginable such as: practice a sport, make love, play a musical instrument, or just enjoy the view. And it all seems so real!

More to the point, the same subconscious mind that designs a dream world can also be tapped into here in the real world because real-life reality also resonates by subconscious design. That's why similar to a lucid dream world, an alignment with a specific frequency of your own real-world subconscious energy – coming from a conscious belief in lucid love – can provide you with some command over real-world subconscious power, the power to control your real-life destiny!

Of course, no one can be as powerful in the real world as a lucid dreamer is in a lucid dream world because there's a "perfect" reason why we won't fully merge with our real-world deeper self. The perfectly real reason why you can't fully merge with your real self is complicated; however, from a Front To Back Thinking point of view… the reason is understandable. First of all, stepping back from a selfish and greedy egotistical attitude enables you to control deeper subconscious power. By comparing subconscious energy in the real world with subconscious energy in a dream world, you may realize how – the same way subconscious energy makes your dream reality feel real – subconscious energy also makes your real-world reality feel real.

While you're sleeping and experiencing a dream world, your dream fantasy can appear – and feel – to be a bona-fide dimension of existence, right up until the point when you wake up. In addition, most folks have flashes of deeper self-awareness during which the real world can appear and feel dreamlike. Just think of a time when you saw a gorgeous sunset with the sky splashed a magical crimson and orange! Or, do you remember ever having come across a candy coloured rainbow? Can you recall how you felt deep down inside of yourself? Did you ever feel like you were in a miraculous, almost dreamlike moment?

More often than not, I'll hear people say that their real-life reality doesn't feel like a good time. An awful lot of people believe that their reality is very disturbing! Similar to remembering good and bad scenes from your real life, you've got good and bad scenes having happened in your dream life too. If you jot down a few quick notes about what was going on, and how you were feeling during any dream, you may easily remember the entire episode. Subconscious energy was the whole "physical" dream along with every good and bad emotion you felt. Unlike the conscious mind, the subconscious mind has no power to think, but it can feel!

Subconscious emotions and physical sensations are also powerful forces of energy in the real world. Consequences of subconscious energy during dream reality and real-life reality are similar in other rational ways too. For instance: when you feel a love for whatever present moment you're experiencing, good things happen! Understanding Lucid Law and the way your subconscious energy works during a dream world enables you to get some control over real-world subconscious energy.

My discovery of the seven lucid laws came from learning how to live longer in a lucid dream world, but they've turned out to be more than just a way to prevent a premature awakening from lucid dreaming. Even though I've only discussed five out of the seven so far, by respecting the lucid laws of Resistance, Love, Tossing Your Burden, Living in the Now, and Belief, you can stay a whole lot safer, healthier, and happier in the real world as well as during dream worlds!

The same as with a real-life scientific view on the Earth's gravitational field conforming with perfectly natural mathematical laws, the lucid laws are perfectly natural too. Being perfectly natural means that Lucid Law doesn't break. The lucid laws are just like the laws of gravity in so much as the Earth's gravitational field doesn't break – if you disrespect gravity, you're the one who can get broken!

Resisting reality in ways that go against the "laws" of gravity can make you suffer. For example: some people – while high on drugs and alcohol – honestly believed that their car could actually fly through the air here in the real world, and many of these people didn't (and many folks still don't) survive such trips. Intoxicated consciousness may ignore the laws of gravity since these levels of self-awareness can lose touch with reality. A respectful, caring, and sober "feel" for a real-world gravitational field can bring you some deeper power to control gravity. Science is all about clear-headed perception, and thanks to believing in science – and loving the idea of airplanes – people really can fly!

Your own harmonious resistance to the Earth's gravitational field of energy enables you to harness the real power of gravitational energy since you have to resist gravity in order to stand up! The same as with gravity, certain natural laws apply to electricity. When you respect the natural laws of electrical energy, you can control electrical power by controlling electrical resistance.

More to the point, if you respect the seven interconnected and meshing lucid laws, then similar to the way any dream is powered, you can power up deeper real-life energy! You can command deeper subconscious power by controlling subconscious energy in a healthy way when you understand Lucid Law. For instance: the Lucid Law of Love meshes with the Lucid law of Belief to reveal how, when you feel good because you consciously believe that your outlook is beautiful, your attitude powers up a healthier perception of the present moment. Along with a healthy attitude, there's no getting away from loving your present moment. That's how you can create a happy mood.

Whether in a dream world or in the real world, a conscious belief of what's going on impresses your subconscious mind with a corresponding mood. This way, an attitude can power up a mood. An attitude acts upon your subconscious energy, and your own energy further influences your attitude! Bad moods go hand in hand with downright antagonized attitudes while good moods are usually a category of harmonious conscious and subconscious energy. The more healthy the mood, the more you harmonize with happiness during any dimension of reality.

Harmony with happiness requires harmony with the subconscious mind. Belief in self-definition needs to include the subconscious mind; otherwise, you can end up suffering through an existence that you truly hate!

Your depth of self-awareness may be limited by the boundaries of unhealthy moods and hateful attitudes. A basic understanding of Lucid Law can help you achieve an attitude that balances your conscious mind with your subconscious mind in a healthy way. While consciously impressing a belief in lucid love upon your subconscious mind, you get some deeper subconscious power to make the real world automatically take you in whatever direction you want to go. New direction unfolds automatically because programmed by conscious belief, the subconscious is automatic – your conscious mind does the thinking.

You're capable of loving your real-world experience. Through a lucidly loving connection with healthy subconscious energy, antagonized attitudes disappear and the same old real-world nightmares don't recur! A lucidly loving outlook may be barely clearer than mud, but don't worry because there's lot's more clarification coming! All seven lucid laws are comparable to the harmony of musical energy. Since Lucid Law is also a significant measure of timing, Lucid Law can be heard – and felt.

## Front To Back Thinking (FTBT)

Proven pearls of wisdom pouring from lucid dreaming can bring you entirely new ways to think about the deeper power of real-world subconscious energy. That's why, while reflecting on the real world from an unconventional Front To Back Thinking (FTBT) viewpoint, a lucidly loving attitude makes your subconscious mind feel a deeper love for your present moment, no matter where you are!

Realized after waking from the <u>Clincher</u> lucid dream described near the end of chapter two, this whole new concept of FTBT brought me new definition for deeper, real-world self-awareness. That's because subconscious power provides energy for deeper self-awareness to hear and feel the real point of existence. The last two lucid laws complete a deeper thinking concept of time, space, perception, and behaviour; then, the real point of all existence and the truest meaning of life become perfectly clear. This all happens through a deeper, real-world presence of mind linking you with deeper subconscious power to hear and feel a love for your present moment.

During a lucid dream, the dreamer is consciously aware of being in a dream world. Lucid awareness also links the lucid dreamer with incredible subconscious power and ongoing enlightenment. Soon to be explained, a really long-lasting lucid dream is capable of returning ultimate subconscious power, ultimate enlightenment, and ultimate failure for the lucid dreamer! A real-world presence of mind is a return from such failure!

A real-world, conscious presence of mind won't ever bring you into a full-on merge with ultimate power or ultimate enlightenment, but such an outlook can give deeper love to your present moment. Giving lucid love powers up subconscious energy in a healthy way because you respect the subconscious mind in a harmonious manner. The same way lucid awareness lasts longer thanks to my respecting even one of the lucid laws, a deeper real-world presence of mind also lasts longer.

Lucid Law also brings about an unconventional view on God. Ah yes, I've said it! I've said the name "God" in the context of a superior being. But, "Oh… my… God," there's no need to freak out! A deeper (and scientific) FTBT view on God is unconventional and is nothing like any religious or mythological description; however, a deeper thinking view on an idea of the equality of "God" is essential to have in place in order to understand the real significance of such belief.

We've got billions of people wondering how anyone can possibly believe in God; at the same time, billions more people are forever amazed at why everyone cannot! In the meantime, the interjection "Oh my God" gets repeated again and again by religious and nonreligious individuals from all around the world. Plus, plenty of people write and type OMG which stands in for interjecting with, "Oh my God." Thanks to personal computers and cell phones, OMG gets sent worldwide in text messages, blogs, tweets, and e-mails.

When people feel powerful emotion – whether happy, sad, or mad – interjections are intended to express such emotion. For example: "Thank God! You're here!" Or: "For God's sake, can you give me a hand here?" Or: "Oh my God, what happened?" Note that such interjections are used universally, in a variety of languages. You can even hear the name of God being spoken over and over again when you listen to the radio, watch television, or take in a movie. So, if you use the interjection "Oh my God" out loud or to yourself, to whom are you really appealing? Exactly who, what, and where is this God? I'm talking about living proof, here and now.

Not so surprising, when individuals attempt to have a mature discussion about who God actually is – or isn't – arguments happen! Questions such as: "Who and what is God?" or "Where could God have come from?" and "Why would God allow so many terrible events to take place here on Earth?" are significant to just about everyone.

If you think about the deeper subconscious power up for grabs with these types of profound questions, how do you feel? Do you have believable answers? Do your beliefs bring you control over your destiny, or do they leave you feeling sort of... lost? A real-world FTBT mindset gets you some deeper subconscious power to redirect your own outlook by enabling you to understand the true purpose for all forms of existence!

Although lucid dreaming and lucid awareness are attainable for some folks, having your own lucid dream is not a necessity for realizing the true purpose of life. A path toward finding the real you – the "One" who can bring about a happy real-world dimension of reality – begins by understanding the way subconscious energy responds to deeper, real-world thinking.

Lucid awareness only occurs during a lucid dream world, but figuring out how Lucid Law works enables you to step into a deeper thinking mindset without having had a lucid dream. Then again, respecting Lucid Law also gives your conscious mind the authority to eventually step into a lucidly aware presence of mind during your own lucid dream.

Whether in a dream world or in the real world, feeling good or bad depends on your mood. The reason a subconscious mood can power heavenly or unsettling dream worlds is simple: whatever you say or do in any dream world, you say and do to your deeper dreaming self. That's why your words and thoughts come back to you in patterns of imaginative subconscious energy that may feel good or bad.

Subconscious moods can also power seemingly heavenly, or disturbing real-world outlooks because just like life in a dream world, real-life reality is also a world of subconscious energy that may feel good or bad. During a dream world, your subconscious mind channels conscious energy via dream souls. Feeling a hateful mood in a dream world means that you're channelling a hateful outlook. That's why you can feel hatred. When you hate the present moment that's taking place during your dream world, you're hating a powerful expression from your own mind, and such energy flies back at you in some form of fear, anger, or hurtfulness. Channel conscious love for your present moment, receive subconscious love and joy in return.

Whether harmonious or inharmonious with how you want to feel, the mood you create within a dream world flows within your dream world's present moment. Your conscious mind directs a rhythmic tuning of subconscious energy that fabricates a dream reality. This means conscious belief loops back at you. You're the "One" creating and living your nightmares as well as good dreams!

The same way the lucid laws of Resistance, Love, Tossing Your Burden, Living in the Now, and Belief relate to dreams and real-world reality, so does the "Lucid Boomerang Law". The Lucid Boomerang Law is also about balancing conscious and subconscious energy. When you understand why whatever you send out verbally, in thought, or in conduct loops back at you like a boomerang, you can believe in the importance of sending lucid love!

The Lucid Boomerang Law is all about understanding the relationship between the power of conscious energy and the power of your own mood in any dimension of reality. For example: if you get yourself into a profound state of anger, you're sending anger into a dimension of existence that you believe to be real. That's why more anger returns to wreak havoc with your subconscious mood; send lucid love, feel more of whatever you believe to be beautiful subconscious energy fly back. If you deceive, you're deceived; if you help, you're helped. Comprehend, feel, and flow with the ideas and understandings arriving with the Lucid Boomerang Law, and any dimension of reality can return a harmoniously joyful mood.

You may easily impress your subconscious mind with lucid love and feel a harmoniously joyful mood. I've talked about harmonious joy, but in order to make this subconscious mood long-lasting, another subconscious impression is necessary – delightful surprise! Delightful surprise is all about feeling astonishment, revelation, awe, and thrill! That's why a delightfully surprising journey into dazzling new personal power is right here, right now, and happens to be in the palms of your hands! By feeling some faith in the deeper power of your own subconscious mind, you may dare to read onward and enter boldly into a fresh frontier, a miraculous presence of mind where you've most likely never been before!

## CHAPTER FOUR

# THE DREAMER

You may want to care about all the different levels of self-awareness that bring your dreams to life. A dream diary is proof that each and every dream soul is you! During a dream, every seemingly individual dream soul – even a tree's subconscious energy – can be admired and respected because you're not superior or inferior to yourself. Showing respect for the equality of all the seemingly individual levels of self-awareness occurring in a dream world returns respect for the dream world's deeper self – you the dreamer.

Caring about difficulties occurring for your levels of self-awareness in dream worlds creates emotional sympathy for the suffering of all dream souls, often with a desire to help; meanwhile, why would you want to care about all the different levels of self-awareness that bring the real world to life? This question takes a while to answer!

A closer look at any dream diary proves how every dream world is a multidimensional mind imagining a space-time continuum that feels real. Once again, the space continuum during a dream world may be understood as being the "physical" fabric of subconscious energy. A dream's time continuum may be identified as being imaginative energy that's self-aware. Subconscious energy doesn't actually think; the subconscious mind is self-aware, is always listening through pure sensation, and has no sense of humour. Not only that, the subconscious "minds" conscious belief.

Consciousness is the thinking part of a person's mind. Remarkably, comparable to every conscious individual in the real world, each conscious individual in a dream world can also feel to be a separate and real self. In a dream world and here in the real world, individuals are the "ones" who live, so there's some legitimacy in believing that consciousness is a separate essence of life, a seemingly separate self. People – and conscious dream souls – often say that "I have a body," or that "I'm in my body." Consciousness feels separate from the physical soul's subconscious energy.

Modern science points me in a similar direction in so far as the part of the mind containing consciousness is called the ego. There's also an assumption that a person's ego is created by the brain in their body's head; however, while in a lucid dream world, a lucidly aware point of view makes me understand that a dreaming mind can have different dream souls channelling different degrees of ego consciousness, all at the same time.

Subconscious energy is a soulful branch because it involves physical energy: it's the fabric for a physical brain, entire body – a person's "heart and soul". An ego comes from points of view acquired through their soul's five senses: sight, sound, touch, taste, and smell. Plus, an ego's conscious attitude arrives through soulful sensations of space, time, and self-awareness. To complete this concept, an ego's attitude makes an impression on their soul's mood. This way, a dream soul exists in a dimension of reality that feels real. As a dream character's attitude impresses their deeper subconscious mind, their soul returns bodily feelings and moods that can create a sensation of the ego being a separate self.

Once more, subconscious energy is self-aware because subconscious energy is a state of mind. For example: a considerate counsellor (or hypnotherapist) often tries to help a client heal their disconnected and troubled ego by working to impress therapeutic beliefs upon the client's subconscious mind. Helping a client toss their selfish and greedy egotistical attitude is what's really happening! An egotistical attitude comes from subconscious energy that's been impressed by conscious belief in superior and inferior levels of self-awareness. Connection with deeper self-awareness can bring conscious and subconscious energy back into balance.

A human baby's physical presence – subconscious soul – originates from a special linking of their mother and father's inner oomph. What I mean is, a newborn may be viewed as being a body of soulful energy.

As with the fabric of all physical energy, soulful energy does whatever it's directed to do. Souls have evolved to automatically make their physical bodies grow, develop, age, and eventually die. Plus, human souls can channel a subconsciously aware time continuum into a conscious level of self-awareness!

This simple description about consciousness emphasizes the idea that subconscious energy can't actually think about stuff. Once again, subconscious energy gets channelled into consciousness through a soul's senses and sensations. An ego can further impress the deeper subconscious mind with a belief in their soul being separate and superior due to their higher education, greater wealth, better gender, finer ethnicity, or their soul's beauty. By the same token, an ego can also impress the subconscious mind with a belief in their soul being separate and inferior due to their lower education, poverty, vulnerable gender, unpopular ethnicity, or their soul's ugliness. Same as in a lucid dream world, a healthy way to love the real-world present moment that you're experiencing – while accomplishing long-lasting survival – is to impress your subconscious mind with conscious belief in the equality of everyone's self-awareness!

An answer to that huge question about why you would want to care about everyone here in the real world begins by understanding the idea that your conscious mind isn't really separate, superior, or inferior since – same as in all dream worlds – self-awareness is the presence of time. All levels of self-awareness are connected because every seemingly separate soul adds depth to the present moment. Insight into the presence of time can make you care about all real-world souls because you may consider how all levels of conscious and subconscious self-awareness add life to the same space-time continuum.

A lucid dream world is a dimension of existence where my lucid level of self-awareness is able to recognize why such existence has a deeper presence of mind powering the lucid dream world's "physical" reality. A deeper level of lucid awareness impresses my dream's space-time continuum with lucid love, tossing fearful feedback in a healthy and natural way. My lucid dream world is impressed with a lucidly loving belief that all souls are equal in value because every degree of self-awareness is a shielded version of the same dreaming self. This way, I automatically release my lucidly aware dream soul from feeling so selfish, greedy, and unhappy!

A link with deeper self-awareness during a lucid dream world brings about my lucidly aware dream soul's more respectful and compassionate attitude. Such a link makes my healthier attitude care for the dream world's present moment by caring about each individual degree of my own self-awareness.

Linking with a good reason to care about the real-world present moment – by understanding why there's also an equality to all real-life souls – helps you toss burdening subconscious energy accompanying real-world selfishness, greed, and unhappiness.

An egotistical attitude comes from a disconnected degree of self-awareness, an outlook that's incapable of comprehending the idea that there's deeper, real-life self-awareness. From an egotistical thinking point of view, you may honestly believe that your ego conscious is a state of mind who's isolated and separate because your body's brain is isolated and separate, but this outlook isn't fully accurate!

## **The Golden Lucid Dream**

The <u>Golden</u> lucid dream started off with me wondering where I was. Though the light was dim, I stood in what appeared to be a huge cavern, seeming to be in what I at first thought was a stone cave because rough rock felt cool to my touch. The air was moist, but smelled clean – I could hear the sound of water gurgling; then, I suddenly remembered everything about my real world.

A light pinch on my right thigh felt dull. I looked down, directly between my feet, took in a deep breath. Even though I was in my late forties, had gained a lot of experience with lucid dreaming, I still felt really excited!

Once I breathed through my excitement, I noticed that my bare feet were on a cool, polished, marble path. After I looked up from the path, the cavern brightened. I could see huge and heavy looking burgundy curtains hanging above stone walls. Glancing at the beautiful curtains, I realized that I wasn't in a cavern at all – I was in an enormous tented building where burbling streams of crystal clear water mingled with fern-rimmed lily ponds.

This tented building was the size of a football stadium. Set high up into what appeared to be a sloped canvas ceiling, giant sized screens were open to the sky, which would brighten and dim due to random clouds passing by. For the time being, some sunshine was beaming down all around me. The pristine water features, flowers, and greenery were bathed in warmth. In addition, many large and highly wrought steel chests bordered the marble path.

I walked along the polished path until I came across a huge chest with it's lid gaping wide open – it was full of gold coins! Of course, I just had to stop and pluck one out. I picked up a big one, in mint condition. The radiant coin felt extraordinarily heavy in my hand. I held this gold coin in my clenched fist while continuing on a slow and cautious walk along the pathway. I kept my other hand free, palm up, and focused on an intention to make this lucid dream bring me my deepest desires – as long as they were harmonious with lucid love!

After walking further along the marble path, I admired several more open chests, which were filled with gemstones, pearls, necklaces, bracelets, rings, golden goblets – all precious items. To boot, the chests themselves were exquisite! They had ornate carvings of animals and birds painted on their jewel studded lids.

Finally, I reached a huge round table that shone like a mirror made from pure silver. The glistening tabletop was spread with all kinds of food. There were large plates of scrumptious looking bread rolls, big bowls of steaming hot soups, dishes filled with vibrant vegetable salads, magnificent platters of multi-coloured fruit, and various types of nuts – all familiar favourites!

I placed my gold coin on the tabletop as a sort of payment; then, I ate a handful of ruby red grapes. I was enjoying the sweet taste when two people – a man and a woman – walked right up to the table and began putting food on their plates. They glanced at me, smiled, and said hello.

I murmured, "Howdy." I also picked up a plate, piled on a steaming hot buttered bread roll, more grapes, and quite a few walnuts. Everything smelled so good that my mouth watered in anticipation as I sat down crosswise from the two.

Between bites of delicious food, I took a closer look at the two dream characters. They appeared to be enjoying their meal. Probably in their late twenties, wearing identical tight-fitting foil outfits, they both looked slim, well-proportioned, and each had spiky blonde hair. With similar facial features, the man was strikingly handsome, but it was the woman who really caught my attention. Her attractiveness had me sitting up straight, shoulders pulled back, chest puffed out, and I'm sure I had a goofy look on my face!

I finally asked: "Are you two related by any chance?" Eating my food as politely as possible, I munched with my mouth shut while waiting for an answer.

The youthful fellow looked up from his plate. After swallowing, he said, "Why yes sir, we are." He waved at the woman beside him with his fork, "This is my sister Samantha, and my name is David."

"Well hello David and Samantha, I'm William. Nice to meet you."

The pair merely nodded. After a slight pause, I asked: "Are you two from around here?"

David set his knife and fork onto the gleaming tabletop, stood in order to reach out and scoop up the nearby gold coin that I'd placed, looked me in the eye and said, "We all come from the essence of mindfulness."

David's response made me rock back in my chair! I stopped munching while staring up at him; then, I chewed really fast – swallowed as quickly as possible.

David seemed to be waiting for another question. He sat back down, and all the while his sister continued eating unhurriedly, bit by bit.

"Uh, hmm… So, you come from the essence of mindfulness? Wow, that sounds really far-out."

"Well, you asked," he said in a voice that sounded sincere.

The pair seemed like an offshoot of the treasure surrounding me, and David's next words confirmed my thought. He said, "I shall answer any question, and Samantha is yours to direct – she shall answer any desire." His straight-faced expression was as solemn as his flat tone of voice.

"Ok." I immediately glanced over at Samantha and found it difficult to take my eyes off her. In my real world, I was no longer married – was single; getting intimate with Samantha would quite likely be the most wonderful treasure of all! Then again, perhaps a philosophical conversation with David might prove to be a new kind of treasure.

I turned my attention back toward David, instantly decided to first discover more about his "answers", and asked: "Hey David, maybe you could explain what you mean by your coming from the essence of mindfulness? What exactly is the essence of mindfulness?"

"The essence of mindfulness is self-awareness."

"Oh yeah, maybe I agree with you there, but where does your mind come from?"

"The essence of a mind is self-awareness, and a person's mind comes from the way their physical body – their soul – channels subconscious energy into conscious energy."

If I didn't know that I was in a dream world, such a reply might've been confusing; however, from a lucidly aware point of view, David's answer made sense. His conscious mind came from the way his "physical" soul channelled a stream of the dreamer's subconscious energy. At this point, I decided I liked the way things were going. David seemed sincere, open-minded, and was kind of friendly.

"If we're channelling subconscious energy, then how come we feel like individuals?" I asked, with a smile.

David continued, "Life is a compilation of energy." His blue eyes seemed to brighten. "And," he said, "everyone adds their own conscious energy to help form a whole new dimension of self-awareness because everyone has beliefs that are dependent upon their own outlooks, moods, and attitudes. Believing that you're a separate self results from the individual focus, perception, interpretation, and hunger going along with a natural drive for your biological body to survive."

David paused and gave me a curious look, as though he were examining my level of self-awareness. I was still in a level of lucid awareness, knew that I was dreaming. I'd an entire "universe" in the palms of my hands, was "Captain" and "Crew" in this imaginative dimension of existence, could do anything I wanted to. Yet, I chose to sit, conserve my energy and listen to an extraordinary "crewmember", one who was another offshoot of my own dreaming mind.

Then, in his easygoing and confident manner, David began to speak again. He said, "Most folks agree with the idea that their self-awareness comes from the brain in their head."

I thought about what he was saying, nodded at him and said, "Almost everyone thinks that their brain creates their self-awareness. And yes, a person's personality seems individual and separate from their physical world."

I knew his self-awareness didn't originate from the brain in his head – David came from a deeper dreaming self: his mind branched from a dreaming mind – a self-aware space-time continuum. The same way most real-life folks believe that each person has an independent brain creating their mind, so do most dream characters. Clearly, in any dream world such belief happens to be inaccurate because every dream character's consciousness branches from the same "One" dreamer. Also, each dream character brings a certain degree of self-awareness to life. Unless lucid, every dream soul is shielded from the dreamer's level of self-awareness.

David's response amazed me! He said, "I've lived a long life, had a happy childhood, wonderful family and friends, but I believe I'm more than just a personality in a body."

Well, he was right. I recognized that there was a lesser amount of shielding involved with David's deeper thinking mindset, and I felt delightfully surprised because unexpectedly, here was the most extraordinary dream character I'd ever met!

David leaned back from the table, folded his hands on his lap, and continued: "Outside, there're large living organisms such as gigantic trees which don't have brains, but there's certainly some sort of self-awareness going on. A tree spreads roots, grows, creates seeds, reproduces, and even dies, but there's no brain. So, where does a tree's spirit of life come from?

I smiled and replied, "That's a good question."

Now I thought it was my turn to answer; nevertheless, I wanted to be careful. There were times when I'd preached to dream characters – tried to lecture about how and why a deeper dreaming self was imagining everyone and everything in an instant of dreamtime. I would try to explain that by loving to be present, we could drive the dream's imaginative energy in a healthier, longer lasting direction.

My trying to give a clear and detailed account of lucid awareness usually caused conscious dream souls to express bewilderment, often followed by snorts of mocking scorn. After my declaring that we were all in a dream world, "they" would inevitably become appalled at my saying so with such sincerity. Enjoying his openness and honesty, I stayed in tune with David by showing deeper respect and compassion for his outlook.

I was still thinking about being respectful with my words when David uttered a most remarkable statement, suddenly saying: "I think a bigger picture on reality opens if we can understand that consciousness is really a protected degree of deeper self-awareness."

Now David really did have me in agreement. That's why I said, "Yes, I believe you're right. All levels of self-awareness come from the same deeper self. There's an inconspicuous equality to everyone. Neither one of us could possibly be superior or inferior to one another because we both branch from the same "One" deeper self. And, this deeper self also exists in another dimension of reality."

David went on in a slightly quicker tone, "So, all self-awareness is everyone's, how did you put it... deeper self?"

My voice was getting calmer as I said, "Ah yes, and our deeper self isn't disconnected from that tree you were talking about. Everything physical is the same deeper and greater self's subconscious mind, and self-awareness is the same deeper self's spirit of life. This way, a tree's spirit of life also branches from the same deeper and universal self. That's why a tree doesn't need a brain to express it's level of subconscious self-awareness."

"You understand!" David finally began to sound excited.

"I suppose I've some extra special ideas and concepts about connecting with a more caring presence of mind." I felt myself grinning at him again and added, "For me, mindfulness is all about a caringly conscious outlook."

He smiled back this time, continued by saying, "Exploring who and what self-awareness – our deeper self – really is, begins by investigating who we believe we are..."

I just had to interrupt, "Wait a sec, a person expresses a different degree of self-awareness than a tree – our level of self-awareness is conscious, seems individual and separate."

"Oh!" said David, "It's the same self that's being channelled, but the medium doing the channelling is what's different. Consciousness, or what the psychology books call "ego", it comes from the way a brain and body channel subconscious energy." He tilted his head towards me and whispered, "A person's reality is normally perceived from an individualistic viewpoint – it feels like we're independent from one another, from the trees, animals, birds and everything, but we're all connected because we're all channelling the spirit of the same self whom you were talking about."

David was on a triumphant roll and his voice picked up in volume with a most wonderful finale: "A deeper level of conscious energy gets powered up from individuals connecting with one another!"

"One more question?" I gazed into his big blue eyes and asked: "What is the spirit of life, and where did it come from?"

David touched his chin with a forefinger. "Oh that's easy to answer. The original spirit of life arrived with the beginning of time – is the present moment."

His answer startled me so much that I was overcome with glorious and giddy wonder! I returned to the real world with an unexpected jolt. On went my bedside light, out came my dream diary, and my account of this Golden lucid dream was written down in detail!

## Glorious Wonder!

My amazement with what I named as being the Golden lucid dream rang with astounding beauty, exhilarating splendour, and glorious wonder! When David said that the original spirit of life arrived with the beginning of time, which was the dream world's present moment, I understood that he meant a measure of time comes from the dreamer's presence of mind!

Eventually, my amazement stabilized while I was writing in my dream diary because I began to question what David might've meant when he said consciousness is really a protected degree of deeper self-awareness. Why is consciousness protected (shielded) from a merge with the dream world's deeper self?

Right then and there, I recognized how and why – from David's point of view – being shielded from a complete merge with lucid awareness was also protecting the dreamer from something which is incredibly significant. Since I was fully merged with my dreaming mind while in that Golden lucid dream's dimension of existence, and thanks to my lucid dream soul's deeper level of lucid awareness, I knew exactly what David's ego was helping to protect the dream world from. In order to put it into words, I just needed to slow down, take my time, and balance a deeper thinking presence of mind with a lucidly loving outlook.

While linked with a deeper thinking presence of mind, the same shield and protection for consciousness is also recognizable right here and now, in the real world! The mystery behind such shielding and protection unravels before the end of the next chapter, after more about Lucid Law gets explained and clarified.

Getting back to the real treasure that I brought home from the <u>Golden</u> lucid dream – the idea that a spirit of life is the present moment made me marvel at how the dreamer could actually come from every dream soul. I'd always assumed that the creator came first, but since every protected level of self-awareness adds more life to the dream world's present moment, the dreamer could actually come from the dream world's present moment because Dreamtime is an expression of self-awareness.

A deeper dreaming self lives "soulful" sensations of existence through each dream soul – concurrently. While a dream unfolds, the dreamer is each dream soul, but how does the time continuum taking place during a dream world connect an individual dream soul with lucid awareness? Expanding conscious belief that all individual levels of self-awareness flow within one greater stream of universal thought helps explain how a dream world's time continuum can connect with lucid awareness: it's all about waking up!

David's idea about an original spirit of life being Dreamtime woke me up! If a deeper and universal dreaming self arises from all the commotion going on in a dream world, I could also look into the idea that a deeper and universal real-world self arises from all the commotion going on in the real world too!

Although the "river of life" during a dream world is more like a "stream of thought", the idea that conscious dream souls energize their own protected streams of thought can be super helpful for understanding more about subconscious power. Similar to each "living" soul in a dream world channelling a time continuum that's streaming within a deeper self's presence of mind, a real-world soul can also be viewed as channelling a time continuum that's streaming within a deeper self's presence of mind.

Whether in a dream world or in your real world, does your ego define who and what you are, or does every ego contribute to a deeper and self-perpetuating stream of thought that defines who and what you are? Same as the way a real river of water can appear to be self-perpetuating for a certain period of time, so can dream worlds. A river doesn't exist just because it's there, it began from an original source that eventually channelled the river. But, a river is always being supplied continuously, may seem unchanging even though it streams from the presence of each water droplet all at once. Dream worlds also stream from the presence expressed by each dream soul, all at once. So, what came first, a stream of thought or an individual presence of mind?

Abruptly, I had a flash of insight – a viable solution to the ancient query about what came first, the chicken or the egg? My answer for the chicken and egg mystery is that the egg came first!

Once again, deeper thinking also links with a scientific viewpoint since a real-world river of consciousness appears to have originated from a primordial pudding. One scientific theory behind evolution is that a "big bang" started everything – which may be thought of as subconscious energy banging into "physical" existence. Eventually, as the ingredients for single celled souls aligned in naturally occurring, egg-like mixtures, different levels of subconscious self-awareness began to hatch. But, there's still the question of where the real-world space-time continuum originally came from?

Same as a dream world, the real-world comes from a deeper, multidimensional mind; along with this idea, the real-world time continuum may be understood as being a universal river of self-awareness. That's because every soul channels a present moment in order to have a level of self-awareness!

A conscious belief in having a good or a bad time impresses your real-world physical soul with good or bad emotion. Such soulful subconscious moods add life to any dimension of existence. Continuing to grow and evolve within a dimension of reality that feels real, your soul can channel the essence of mindfulness – a more caring level of deeper self-awareness – into the real world, instantly.

This important idea about a deeper presence of mind banging the real world into existence means that every real-world soul is connected with a universal self, and that's why a soul's level of self-awareness can transform. The real universe banged into existence the same way dream worlds bang into existence – with miraculous instantaneousness, a self-perpetuating existence being protected by shallower levels of self-awareness.

More to the point, while you live and breathe, you can toy with a conscious belief that similar to every dream world, a river of conscious and subconscious energy is the real world! From my Golden lucid dream, David gave an answer for deeper self-definition when he said that "The essence of a mind is self-awareness, and a person's mind comes from the way their physical body – their soul – channels subconscious energy into conscious energy."

David also said that "A deeper level of conscious energy gets powered up from individuals connecting with one another!"

During the same instant that a dream world is happening, the dreamer is every degree of self-awareness – the dreamer is every seemingly separate individual in the dream world, all at the same time. The conscious self-awareness that a dream character channels from the dream world's present moment is the dreamer's presence of mind. Just like the way a river of water gets channelled by the deeper terrain beneath it, consciousness gets channelled by deeper terrain – subconscious self-awareness. The real river of life has a conscious connection too, and that's why deeper subconscious power returns to a real-world soul who's linked with lucid love. Giving lucid love makes consciousness mindful of a present moment being self-aware!

The same way the dreamer is usually overlooked, forgotten, and denied by dream characters, a deeper and universal real-world self is usually overlooked, forgotten, and denied by most real-world souls; however, while bringing conscious and subconscious energy into balance via a lucidly loving and deeper thinking outlook, a new and unconventional view on self-definition emerges. That's because a universal, real-world self – a presence of mind that comes from all real-world conscious and subconscious levels of self-awareness, all at the same time – emerges, automatically. Now, you may begin to believe the idea that your ego is like a "droplet" of consciousness who's flowing within one greater river of universal thought!

## Ego Consciousness

Throughout the ages, entire cultures have had (and still have) many different ideas, theories, and thoughts about how the universe began to flow. There've been all sorts of discussions, arguments, and fights over the differences in people's opinions on this subject! Even in lucid dream worlds, questions about how such a dimension of reality began are sometimes raised by conscious dream characters. As I mentioned earlier, I've experienced episodes of lucid awareness during which I preached on all existence being connected with a deeper presence of mind, only to be ignored or ridiculed by fellow dream characters.

In hindsight, I recognize why my preaching without a compassionate explanation contravened guidance from Lucid Law. That's because such sermons didn't respect a dream character's point of view. Trying to expand an awareness of what's really going on can be a tumultuous experience, just ask any counsellor! If the truth behind a belief in self-definition gets challenged in a sudden way, powerful feelings of fear and uncertainty may unexpectedly rush through the subconscious mind, and the resulting mood won't feel nice.

A healthy and rational view on a deeper meaning of all existence can arrive by discovering the way lucid awareness and a dream world's deeper self connect. This way, a subconscious mind can easily accept the new and more daring idea that connectivity exists for all levels of self-awareness here and now in the real world too.

Once again, lucid love is all about believing that you're connected with your present moment. New awareness of a deeper self being the real world present moment might shake you to the core; nevertheless, you may honestly care about all of real-life reality by loving your present moment. That is, you may begin to love the idea of there being a universal self.

Consciously believing that the present moment is the presence of a universal self gets you some deeper subconscious power to create a long-running good mood. That's because a conscious belief in new self-definition is an example of a life changing world view. So, get ready to have some of your old world views challenged in healthy ways!

A multidimensional mind can bang new dimensions of dream reality into existence; although, dropping this concept onto my consciously aware dream characters wasn't winning me any popularity contests. That's why the real challenge is to slow down, toss over-excitement, and really think!

Even though there've been dream characters who were interested in my revelations, before I could ever finish explaining myself, most would react with total disbelief! Challenging another's belief can be dangerous. Fellow dream characters would often become unfriendly, then angrily proclaim me to be ridiculous for even suggesting such a preposterous idea that all souls come from the same dreaming mind!

Any dimension of reality that's created and expressed by a deeper presence of mind has a purpose. There's also a deeper purpose for having an ego: it's to do with survival, but it's for the survival of a universal self. When you understand more about lucid awareness, you can transform unhealthy truth behind belief in self-definition, stir up a lucidly loving attitude and realize a far greater outlook through your own compassionate window of self-awareness.

Again, a deeper thinking mindset can reveal not only how dream characters channel consciousness through sight, sound, touch, taste, and smell – a conscious dream soul also gives rise to some basic sensations: space, time, and self-awareness. Every sense and sensation becomes important when analyzed singly, and each contributes to the dreamer's greater stream of multidimensional thought.

During dream worlds and in the real world, conscious belief gets impressed upon the subconscious mind, and a world view conforms to a reality that feels real. A lucidly loving attitude can get you some deeper subconscious power in dream worlds and here in the real world because parallel with a conscious belief that all souls are linked with a universal self, a healthier world view arrives. Loving whatever space-time continuum you're helping make feel real brings you a lucidly loving outlook, a real-world view where you get some deeper subconscious power to take your own attitude in whatever direction you want to go!

While realizing that your attitude has an effect on your subconscious mood, and your subconscious mood has an effect on your attitude, you can feel lucid love transforming the idea that your ego is a superior (or inferior) level of self-awareness. Through a lucidly loving attitude, you're capable of feeling compassion and respect for everyone because similar to every soul in a dream world, you may view every real-life soul as being your deeper self, and therefore of equal value.

Belief in immortality during a lucid dream world comes from trusting that a dreamer imagines and lives the entire dream world. I can merge with a deeper level of lucid awareness because channelling is a two-way street. During any dream world, the dream souls channel dream life instantaneously, and at the same time the dreamer lives dream life through each dream soul. When I know I'm dreaming and consciously believe that I'll eventually return to my real-life home, I won't believe that any soul's death is the end of that soul's life. Amazingly, without a fear of death, my happiness surges significantly! Linking with lucid awareness while in a lucid dream world creates conscious belief in a universal self being the dream world. That's because each dream soul channels the presence of the same "One" dreamer.

So, a deeper thinking person who's balanced with a lucidly loving outlook might ask a real-life hot dog vendor: "Please, can you make me one with everything?"

But seriously, before you can consciously believe that you're "One" with an immortal real-life self, a step back into the murk may be necessary. Taking a good look at the fearful moods a disturbed subconscious mind can drag you through reveals why you may really suffer from too much fear, anger, and hurt in your dream life, not to mention your real life!

## Ego, And Egotism

I like to describe the human ego as a branch of conscious energy that streams from a feisty spirit to survive. An ego gets channelled by a subconscious sensation of what feels real. To facilitate this new idea about conscious energy being channelled into existence, you may consider how every dream character is part of a greater subconscious mind.

Subconscious energy is your body, which includes an ever evolving brain, eyes, ears, nose, tongue, "heart", and everything else helping you to perceive your unique point of view. This way, not only does your ego consciously impress your soul with whatever you believe to be real, your physical soul impresses your consciously aware ego by means of physical and emotional sensation.

For most folks, their subconscious mood gets expressed through their conscious attitude. For example: an old square rigged sailing ship was cruising past a remote tropical island when a crew-member spotted three huts and a man who'd been stranded there for many years. The captain sent a party of sailors ashore to rescue the castaway.

After the initial excitement of the rescue, one of the sailors asked the castaway: "So, what's that there first hut for?"

"That's me wee house," said the castaway.
"What's the second hut for?"
That's me wee church."
"And the third hut?"
Oh that?" sniffed the castaway, "That's the church I used to go to."

Egotistical attitudes can make you a type of castaway. With a selfishly proud belief in your soul's ego being superior to that of another soul's ego, you can cause your soul to be cast far adrift because whatever you consciously believe also carries deeper emotional consequences.

Rescuing a disconnected ego from being cast further adrift by their belief in superior and inferior levels of the same self-awareness can have you streaming with deeper subconscious power – the subconscious power you get from giving lucid love. Hot dog! This is one great way to feel optimistic about there really being a universal meaning to everyone's life!

A willingness to expand your ego into a less guarded level of consciousness can broaden and deepen the definition of your own self-awareness. Similar to having lucid awareness during a lucid dream world, you may go so far as to first deliver an insight, then a recognition, and finally a conscious understanding of how you're always connected with a universal self – while "wide" awake! This way, you may believe that a universal self is "One" with everything.

## Taking A New Path

When I was a young man, I often felt insignificant and trivial whenever I contemplated on the momentous dimension of real-life reality. That is, I felt totally lost while trying to understand a deeper meaning behind my own comparatively infinitesimal body of life. Through a chronic and exhaustive belief in being insignificant and trivial compared to all of real-life reality, you may also feel lost when contemplating on a truer meaning of life.

You may implode and fall flat if you believe in a physical measure of existence, instead of understanding what you're actually trying to measure – your subconscious mind. You can get marooned in a dimension of measurement – a place where belief in physical isolation is directly proportional to your soul's distress!

The branch to a limitless, deeper, and universal presence of mind gets forgotten, ignored, and eventually denied by an ego who remains contracted with egotistical thinking. Any glimpse at a truer meaning of life gets blurred by conscious belief in self-definition being a physical measurement. A belief in physical measurement defining your sensation of self-awareness lacks the inclusiveness of universal self-awareness, whereas a deeper thinking mindset can help you understand how the physical world is made of subconscious energy. Belief in your own subconscious mind being multidimensional – because you can instantly imagine a dream world – makes it possible to connect your ego with a different attitude. This different attitude tunes you into the idea of flowing with – and being one with – a universal self.

Along with healthy truth behind belief in a deeper, universal self being everyone, and a universal subconscious mind being everything, your ego is capable of impressing your own soul with a different identity. Instead of feeling lost when contemplating on a deeper meaning of life, you may always feel connected with everyone and everything. Unsettling moods may be tossed when you understand why your ego is an expression of deep significance.

A lucid dream world appears to be real, yet, I believe that such a dimension of reality is truly an illusion. This perception occurs because with lucid awareness in place, I'm able to remember my entire real-world reality. Even though a lucid dream world feels real, I believe that such a dimension of reality is an imaginative illusion taking place within my own mind. That's because simultaneously, I'm the creator and the creation. A definition of lucid awareness can't be based on physical measurement. A deeper thinking and lucidly loving, real-world mindset makes me understand that the real world is also an imaginative illusion!

A competitively tough level of egotistical thinking – destined for a belief in superior and inferior levels of self-awareness – may freeze into place if you believe in a measurement of self-worth. Egotistical thinking can measure and compare your physical appearance, social standing, and mental competence against perfection!

Astrophysicists work to come up with perfect mathematical formulas to help measure and describe the different types of energy flowing in the real world. As far as energy goes, the universe may seem to stream forth with the perfection of mathematical measure; however, the universe can also be living proof of perfect imperfection when it comes down to putting a measure on your level of self-worth!

A computer program expresses perfect mathematical measure and can measure up as a superior state of artificial intelligence. But, a computer hasn't got any self-awareness because it lacks a spirit of life. A computer program is capable of counting really fast, but doesn't actually feel the present moment. That's why artificial intelligence is incapable of dreaming. A spirit of life is more than just a measurement of time, a spirit of life is time. Genuine consciousness is a present moment. Clearly, there's a danger of spinning in dizziness while trying to balance conscious and subconscious energy with physical measure; meanwhile, a quick look at a most amazing period of human history helps connect a level of ego conscious with a deeper state of mindfulness.

## Good, And Evil

There was an ancient Greek period during which many Athenian citizens believed in Mount Olympus, and that a group of gods lived there. Zeus was considered to be most powerful, even though all the gods were thought to have superior levels of self-awareness. During this amazing period of human evolution, a new philosopher became well known. Historians tell us how Socrates (469-399 B.C.) asked: "What's the difference between good, and evil?"

Fellow Athenians replied, "The gods judge what's good, and what's evil."

Talking about Socrates is pertinent at this point in the development of deeper mindfulness because even though his story took place over 2400 years ago, you may understand why superior levels of self-awareness could have seemed perfectly true for an Athenian. You may also realize the folly with such belief! The Delphic Oracle of Apollo was one of the most famous ancient shrines where people could go to consult a priest or priestess during times of trouble; messages believed to have come from a god in response to a request, plea, or petition were handed down.

Socrates raised many questions designed to have Athenian citizens come up with their own clear and concise answers (his manner of questioning was a big part of his claim to fame). In answer to some of his publicly probing query, Socrates made many Athenian's realize how, according to the oracles, a god might proclaim that someone's exploit – such as a war – was good, while another god might proclaim that the same exploit was evil.

Through his open manner of questioning, Socrates had Athenians understanding that – according to the differing decrees coming from various gods – the same person and their exploit might be judged as good by one god, evil by another. In brief, because everyone agreed that there was a definite difference between good, and evil, there was no way that a person could be both good and evil at the same time. So, some Greek gods must sometimes be wrong!

Greek history shows how Socrates led the Greek empire along a path of tremendous upheaval and change. That any god could make a mistake meant a trust in their rulings might also breakdown. That's why Socrates was sentenced to death!

Socrates probably knew there was danger involved with trying to transform a person's belief, let alone that of an empire! A world view can be flung into disorder if the subconscious mind fills with bodily fear coming from a long-established belief – such as the idea of a superior god – being brought into serious question by the ego.

From a balanced outlook – good, and evil are ideas. The same as with conscious belief in beauty and ugliness being real, an outlook can feel either harmonious with a belief in beauty (beautiful and good), or harmonious with a belief in ugliness (ugly and evil). The real difference between good, and evil is all about an idea, where "good" conscious energy arrives with a beautiful idea, while "evil" conscious energy arrives with an ugly idea!

For an individual or for an empire, the power of truth behind belief is proportional to the disruption taking place as the idea collapses; nevertheless, an opportunity to balance conscious energy with subconscious energy arrives because a person may take a new path toward a healthier truth behind belief in the equality of conscious energy!

Belief in an objective real-world outlook that's based on facts rather than thoughts or opinions may make you avoid asking powerful questions about a truer meaning of life. Fear from long-established belief in the superiority of beauty and the evil of ugliness can keep varying degrees of unhealthy truth frozen in place, denying you a closer connection with belief in the idea that every individual soul has an equally live connection with deeper subconscious power.

If you overlook, forget, ignore, and deny wisdom pouring from your own dreaming mind, you may believe that your sensation of self-awareness is created by your brain. You may keep going in unhealthy directions by going along with an egotistical outlook that makes you feel: selfish, greedy, unhealthy, and unhappy.

How can you gain some sort of control, keep your ego healthy and happy in a real world that feels more like a perfectly good idea? Here's one answer: power up subconscious energy that's harmonious with lucid love – believe in the idea that everyone's self-awareness is equal in worthiness and significance.

Control over deeper subconscious power arrives from believing in – thereby feeling – a loving connection with a deeper self. Clearly, every dream soul's deeper self is the same – you the dreamer. You experience your dream world through every dream soul during a present moment of "Dreamtime". Existence happens to be similar in the real world because there turns out to be a present moment that's connecting everyone's level of self-awareness here and now, in a real-life space-time continuum!

CHAPTER FIVE

# ETERNITY AND THE MOMENT

At this point in the quest to feel long-lasting happiness that's harmonious with a balanced mind, a peek at how space and time take place during any dream world can illustrate what's going on with space and time in the real world. A space-time continuum is a space and time coordinate system consisting of three spatial coordinates and one for time, in which it's possible to locate events. Since the space-time continuum taking place during a dream replicates the real-world space-time continuum, these words "space" and "time" are really important ideas!

Aside from the fact that a dream world doesn't take up any real-life space, a dream's time continuum is often out of sync with the real-world time continuum. Along with many sunrises and sunsets, my lucid dreams can seem to last for several days, weeks, months, sometimes years! But, according to my bedside clock, every lucid dream takes place in mere minutes of the real-world reality that we all share. Clearly, there's a deep significance to the idea of space and time during every dimension of existence.

In order to answer this question about why there can be a time continuum disparity between a dream world and the real world, you've got to first examine your own idea of "time". If you want to get some deeper subconscious power to manage a long-lasting good time, you need to realize why a belief in conventional linear time – a system for measuring intervals of limited periods during which stuff happens – "happens" to be at odds with a deeper thinking view on the definition of time.

Conforming to socially accepted customs, conscious belief in the idea of time being linear happens to be based on measurements coming from clocks and calendars. Ah yes, back to deep-rooted, physical measurement matters! You can count seconds, minutes, hours, days, and years having passed or which are about to pass, due to the earth's steady spin around the sun. This way, an established belief about a past and a future can conform to the conventional concept that time is a measure. But really, what are the seconds and minutes measuring? A measure of spins the earth makes around the sun? A measure of direction? A measure of the meantime?

Because the conventional concept of time treats "time" as a commodity, a proportionally changing measurement of the Earth's movement around the sun can make you believe that your real-world dimension of time must be linear since never-ending numbers are capable of being represented by a straight line on a graph. But, by comparing a ticking clock with an awareness of the present moment, you may understand how the ticking measures a present moment.

Many scientists agree with the theory that the universe began with a big bang, as I described in the previous chapter. The popular "Big Bang" theory – that the explosion of a single mass of matter started the universe – represents a fantastic notion; however, even this theoretical beginning of time has another mystery due to the constant question: "Where did the single mass of matter come from?"

There's also my idea about the Big Bang theory depicting an additional parallel between real life and dream life, owing to the way dream worlds seem to suddenly, out of nothingness, just bang to life! A dream world arrives with an explosion of expanding subconscious energy. A dream world is a subconscious space continuum that's connected by a subconsciously aware time continuum. Not only that, a dream world's subconscious time continuum can be channelled into conscious self-awareness. A dream world's time continuum – Dreamtime – is the dreamer's subconscious and conscious awareness of an imaginary world in which it's possible to locate events.

Since you may believe that a dream fantasy materializes due to a sudden increase in energy beating within your own multidimensional mind, you might also want to think about how a greater multidimensional mind could also have materialized real-life reality with a similar sudden and energetic big bang beginning! This way, the popular Big Bang theory's single mass of matter may be understood to be a greater subconscious mind. That's why the presence of time is another parallel link with the presence of subconscious self-awareness in the real world, as well as in dream worlds.

Because you may consciously believe that a measurement of time feels real, a problematic attitude can step forward since you may forget about what you're measuring! An ego may believe that an infinite amount of time reaches as far forward as backward since numbers are never-ending. The idea of being at the centre of an infinite time continuum includes a surreal, dreamlike scale of measure. That's because conscious belief in time being linear can have you moving out of a past, into a future, along a forward flow of linear measure.

A view of time being a forward flow of linear measure can also make you believe that linear time trails with separate segments where, for example, a distinct era such as the ancient Greek empire occurred in history. Or, on a smaller scale, an employee's "time" on the job may be divided into separate segments, and the worker can receive an hourly wage for time "spent" on the job.

From people earning a certain amount of money per hour, receiving a monthly salary, celebrating a birthday, or calculating a civilization's life span, belief that the present moment is linear can lead to belief in separate moments of time. That's why so many people seem to believe that time is a measure of direction, with the path of direction being out of a past, and into a future. In other words, belief in your own presence being a physical measurement may cause you to perceive time as being the number of seconds, minutes, hours, days, months or years that have elapsed or are about to elapse. Instead, time is really a self connecting instantaneousness. Wow! What in the world is a self connecting instantaneousness? No worries, it's easy to understand from a deeper thinking point of view.

A perception of time as being linear can cause you to overlook, forget, and deny a conflicting actuality – time is now! Believing that time is linear can deny a lucidly loving outlook because you may ignore the present moment. Contrary to a belief in "time" being a commodity coming from a clockwork of ticking seconds, with each second going by, getting used up and eventually running out, a deeper thinking concept of time turns out to be something else altogether!

Measuring the real-world present moment with clocks and calendars can create belief in an infinite amount of measure. Belief in time being an infinite measure of ticking seconds – instead of understanding that time is a present moment – can create a feeling of time passing by. In actuality, a seemingly individual soul streams within a persistent and perpetual present moment – real-world self-awareness. An awareness of your own presence "passes by" because self-awareness is the essence of time!

Being attentive and feeling the present moment means that you may also get some deeper subconscious power from the ideas and understandings going along with the Lucid Law of Living in the Now. For instance: the idea that time is a self connecting instantaneousness means that the present moment during a dream world is your deeper self's instantaneous connection with all levels of self-awareness in the dream world. That's because your dreaming self is every dream soul's real self.

You may recognize why a presence of mind is central for a dream world's existence. Recognizing that you're at the centre of a time continuum with a past behind you – a future ahead – makes apparent why this "centre" is the presence of subconscious and conscious energy. From this point of view, showing respect for the present moment can change your direction of thought. By focusing on the one instantaneous moment that you're in, you can get a more accurate feel for real time actually being a presence of mind.

The Lucid Law of Living in the Now is different from the Lucid Law of Love because the Lucid Law of Love is all about how deeper love feels: it's about loving to feel present. The Lucid Law of Living in the Now is about understanding why the present moment during any dream arrives with a dreaming mind banging a new dimension of reality into existence, and this important concept helps guide the conscious mind into an awareness of deeper subconscious power!

Many folks seem to think that a time machine might take a person back (or forward) in the measure of time; however, a deeper thinking mindset won't harmonize with such imbalance. It's your subconscious memory that retains impressions of events. That's why, in a manner of speaking, you may travel back through your subconscious memory. Yet, when a person uses their imagination to reminisce on belief in fearful, angry, or hurtful past events, a heartrending mood may arrive. Dwelling on a past (or a future) dread can also channel a fearsome present moment!

Intentionally recalling happy memories in order to keep going in a healthy direction through life is something else altogether. Joyful memory can channel conscious love for the present moment. For example: using your imagination to picture a favourite pet – such as a dog or a cat – can return tender emotion from memory of the pet's personality, enabling a bad attitude to transform into a good one.

By realizing how former emotions can return, you may recognize why channelling love for your present moment is so important! Future emotions depend upon your present attitude. From a deeper thinking outlook, you can learn to love rather than fear your subconscious memories. That's because you can use your imagination to clarify a past event through a lucidly loving point of view. For instance: if a certain perfume reminds you of a lost love and the heartbreak you once felt, an act of forgiveness for the nasty subconscious memory can transform the hurtful mood being triggered by such a scent. Loving your subconscious memory is interconnected with the "Lucid Law of Forgiveness" since an attitude of forgiveness is also a lucidly loving attitude.

The idea behind the Lucid Law of Forgiveness illustrates an important concept about measurable benefit you get from showing forgiveness for an unhealthy truth behind a belief. When you forgive your subconscious mind for having nasty memories, you're harmonious with good returns pouring into your present moment. This act of pardoning unhealthy truth behind belief helps make you pay attention to your present mood. Showing forgiveness goes hand in hand with the all important Lucid Law of Belief, enabling you to feel the forgiveness that you show. You can really only go "back" in memory – the past won't change, but your present and future sure can!

As promised, you're set for a leap in enlightenment because the Lucid Law of Forgiveness is the seventh and final Lucid Law for long-lasting consciousness! The Lucid Law of Forgiveness is all about forgiving yourself. That is, you can forgive yourself for going down paths of selfishness and greed. The Lucid Law of Forgiveness is also about forgiving your deeper self for always experimenting, often flirting with disaster.

From a deeper, compassionate point of view, subconscious memory doesn't come from separate segments of "real" time. A good way to achieve a more forgiving outlook is to realize the concurrent connection between all levels of self-awareness and the "One" present moment. There are no separate periods of time. There aren't any old moments or new moments because there aren't any separate breaks; there's only "One" instantaneous expanse of a perpetual "now".

While the present moment is perceived as a linear measurement, a person can imagine a past and a future; then, a physical measurement of the present moment can create belief in a past and a future. Although you require intelligence to realize such a concept as time being linear, the idea that linear time is a measurement of imagination during one instantaneous moment of existence enables you to perpetuate a healthier level of seemingly separate self-awareness.

A measure of the real-world present moment "goes by", can be bought or spent like a commodity because the measure may be old or new. Measurement has separation points. For example: you can spend some measured "time" working toward a payday.

The universal "One" present moment manifests a living now; nevertheless, an ego may be dominated by conscious belief in a disconnected measure of the present moment as being real time. A party crashing problem with belief in a linear measure of the one present moment being real time involves the infinite decrease. That is, the smallest span of measure can always be cut in half. So, measurement goes the other way too! Even a nanosecond can be halved over and over again. There's no finish to the tiniest amount of linear time because just as you can never reach infinity, a zero measurement of time doesn't exist either. That's because just like the subconscious mind – the presence of self-awareness is beyond measure.

This new view on the contradictory nature of the relationship between linear time and the present moment was discovered by questioning time disparities taking place between dream life and real life. I've more ideas about why measurement of time in a dream world can be out of sync with measurement of time in the real world, but what about space?

## Space

In real life as well as in dream life, a measurement of the three-dimensional expanse where matter exists (appears to exist in a dream world) can go both ways too – physical measurements may be infinitely large or infinitesimally tiny!

Quantum electrodynamics and the "particle zoo" reveal how the tiniest particles can be infinitesimally miniscule. Not only that, physicists have discovered that the same particle can be in different places at the same time! Clearly, there's a measurement problem! That's because imagination is beyond measure. What's more, you can gaze into the grass roots of a dream fantasy and realize another world of infinitesimal particles, or you can look upward into your dream's night sky, and the number of stars may appear to be as infinite as in the real universe!

Unmistakably, a dream world's "physical" reality can be infinitesimally microscopic or infinitely huge. A dream's space continuum is the dreamer's subconscious mind, and every dream soul's shielded sensation of self-awareness adds more depth to their dream world's present moment. As I suggested earlier, self-awareness isn't created by a dream soul's brain, deeper self-awareness is actually shielded by a dream soul's brain. A conscious dream character's brain, heart and soul – subconscious mind – channels a shallower level of the dreamer's self-awareness, helping to perpetuate a different outlook for the dreamer.

Your own conscious mind may now realize the idea that similar to the way a dimension of dream reality bangs into existence, the real universe also banged into existence! That's right, the present space-time continuum is also a self connecting instantaneousness, arrived with an explosion of expanding subconscious energy. Real-life reality is a space continuum that's connected by a time continuum, in which it's possible to locate events.

Since you may believe the idea that a dream world materializes due to a sudden increase in energy beating within your own subconscious mind, you might also want to think about how and why real-life reality originally materialized with a sudden and energetic big bang beginning. That's because by understanding how and why the real universe is a subconscious mind, you can show sympathy for the suffering of others by forgiving any unhealthy truth behind conscious belief. Thanks to a forgiving attitude, you can turn yourself around! The Lucid Law of Forgiveness is all about redefining self-awareness by way of redirecting your own destiny!

## The Essence Of Self-awareness

The essence of self-awareness – your present moment – isn't created by your brain. The present moment is an expression of subconscious energy – the real-life universe. Every brain, heart, and seemingly individual soul channel the same time continuum. What's more, similar to a dream world, the real-world space-time continuum also demonstrates how everybody is linked with an infinitely deep power source since such a dimension of existence feels so real. Once again, there's a real point to a compassionate view on space and time. This point, soon to be defined, is all about the truest meaning of life!

Measurement problems come from a belief in physical measurement. That's why the same particle may appear to be in more than one place at the same time. When it comes down to measurement, there can be problems. For example: during a dream world, the dreamer is everywhere – all at the same time. Thanks to the many different viewpoints of the dream world's souls, the same deeper self is in different places at the same time. And it's the same deal here in the real world where self-awareness is in different real-world places at the same time. Whether subconscious or conscious, live energy is a momentary presence of mind who's every One, everything, and everywhere, all at once. All levels of conscious and subconscious energy are powered by the One present moment.

Paying attention to the mood you're tapped into here in the real world can give you some control over universal subconscious energy because you may now recognize whether or not your mood is harmonious with lucid love. In order to link with lucid love, you need to understand that your own brain, heart, and soul – real-world body – channel a presence of self-awareness. As your real-world space continuum connects your soul with a universal subconscious mind, your real-world time continuum connects your ego with subconscious power. This way, you may recognize time as being a self connecting instantaneousness!

Since a dream world is powered by your own multidimensional mind, you may understand how a presence of mind brings the dream to life.

Self-awareness flows within the dream world's space continuum from many different points of view, all at the same time – while the dream is happening. Valuing the self connecting instantaneousness of your dream souls' experiences enables you to view a deeper self flowing in real-life reality too. This way, you can understand that the real-world space continuum is impressed by what you consciously believe!

Because there's no top, bottom, or any boundaries to the physical size of a dream world while it's happening, a conscious sensation of space and time may seem surreal while you're there. Similar to a dream world, the real-world's three-dimensional expanse – in which all matter really does seem to exist – also appears to contain a cosmic amount of expanding volume. Not only does there seem to be a never-ending amount of space being taken up by real-life reality, there's also your real-life present moment to be accounted for. That's why, similar to a dream world, an endless dimension of a real-life cosmic universe may also seem surreal for your ego.

A measurement of your direction within a real-life, self connecting instantaneousness helps you keep track of what's going on, but when you can understand how real-life reality occurs during one existing instant, you can begin to see why infinity and eternity are simply the here and now. That's how and why, here and now is the time to believe in loving the present moment!

## **Time**

Another time bending perception involves the sensation of how long an event can seem to take. A classic example is waiting for the kettle to boil. When you focus on a good kettle of water, the three minutes that the water takes to boil can feel more like forever!

Then again, while super busy, you may check a clock and feel amazed because several hours "went by" when you felt as though not even one had passed – "time" can seem to have sped up. More importantly, most of us share this same sensation of time flying when we're busy, and crawling when we're bored.

So, just what exactly is boredom? Does boredom alter your sensation of time, or does living through a constant repetition of the same event make you feel tired and slightly annoyed by what at first seemed interesting, entertaining, or exciting? From a deeper thinking viewpoint, boredom's impact on your subconscious mind is super important!

While loving to be in the moment, you can hit the baseball when up to bat, return the sliced tennis ball your opponent skimmed over the net, or even catch the cup you bumped – before it spills. That's because while loving the present moment, you're in control of deeper subconscious power.

Giving love to the living "now" brings you deeper subconscious power to make time seem to slow down; however, if time slows down too much, you may feel a deathlike dullness. For instance: have you ever been in a presence of mind where you felt so bored that you could've died? Most of us have. Resistance to boredom makes you a livewire!

Boredom turns out to be incredibly important because feeling bored means that there's no interesting, exciting, or entertaining novelty happening for you. Your ego can strain with tedium and monotony, create a disapproving attitude, and a wish to change it; besides, this strain isn't harmonious with lucid love since you aren't loving your present moment.

Lucid Law is all about guiding conscious energy in a healthy direction. When you feel bored, you're left with an emptiness – you have deeper subconscious power, but no spirit to feel a love for life. The Lucid Law of Resistance reveals that feeling a love for the present moment can short-circuit from an ego-conscious who's grounded too deeply in boredom. That's why a stable resistance to boredom is a requirement for feeling happy!

While linking a dream world with my real-life ego, my ego passes through a non-resistant phase as I focus on the ground between my feet, and this non-resistant phase feels very calm. Here, in the depths of calmness, I connect with the deeper power of my subconscious mind. After passing through the non-resistant phase, my stable resistance to the deeper boredom I felt from staring at the ground between my feet enables my stable level of lucid awareness to keep the lucid dream world's time continuum alive. While transitioning into lucid awareness during a lucid dream world, the merge with my deeper presence of mind unlocks deeper subconscious power for my lucid level of self-awareness to play with – that's because I feel no fear of death.

Deeper subconscious power can be a challenge to control because even though I want to feel my subconscious mind's power, I don't want to continue feeling bored. But, I do need to continue focusing on the ground between my feet in order to "ground" my surge of overexcited conscious energy. That's why a temporary, non-resistant level of self-awareness makes my attitude calm down. A more relaxed and uncaring realization of being in a dream world links the lucid dreamer with a deeper, more powerful presence of mind. With less resistive energy, I gain more subconscious power! This type of subconscious power impresses my conscious mind with such a huge flash of self-awareness that I can open the door to a whole new dimension of reality... a lucid dream world!

Whew! That was an easy explanation about something that can be difficult to understand. There's more clarification to come, but for now, let's leap out of boredom (thank goodness) and once again focus on the concept of long-lasting lucid dream worlds. Since most dreams begin after going to sleep, and can end before or even while waking up, dream worlds still take place within a real-world present moment. In other words, whether in a dream or in the real world, different measures of the same presence of mind take place during "One" universal present moment called "now".

Conscious belief in the idea of time being linear may make you feel as though some dreams seem to last way longer than the measurements made by your bedside clock. Yet, a lucid dream has me aligned with deeper subconscious power. During a lucid dream world, I can come across a spectacular sunrise and have the morning continue into a full day's worth of events while everything actually happens in mere minutes – according to my bedside clock!

A lucid dream's time continuum being out of sync with my real-world time continuum proves to me that while I'm in a lucid dream world, I'm linked with a different presence of mind than when in the real world. This happens to be another explanation as to why the presence of time in a dream world can be out of sync with the presence of time in the real-world. While linked with lucid awareness, a more detailed and longer lasting "expansion" of the present moment can be maintained and experienced. My dreaming mind expands, speeds up in frequency, or may be said to resonate (molecular theory and quantum physics jargon) at a higher harmonic rate compared to when I'm in the real world.

The real world and dream worlds happen during a present moment. Every dimension of reality is a dimension of space being fabricated by subconscious energy. Self-awareness can resonate out of synch from – but still be part of – real-life reality's time continuum. Not only that, while you're sleeping, your dreaming mind can expand so far into non-resistance that no fantasy appears, no apparent existence takes place – there's no perceptible space, and no present moment seems to be happening. That's because with no resistance, subconscious power peaks. Along with a peak in power, the subconscious mind is completely consenting!

Tranquil conscious resonance within your own sleeping soul explains why many measured hours of real-world reality can vanish from your viewpoint in what feels like no time at all. You feel no resistance to anything. So, who (and where) is your ego while in this tranquil and completely consenting presence of mind?

While your soul is asleep, there's a period where your ego conscious is no longer being channelled! While the conscious part of your mind is turned off, your physical body can connect with the restorative power of your subconscious mind. Subconscious power also helps heal the conscious mind by powering up a world of imaginative existence – a dream world! This way, a dream fantasy makes dream souls perceive a world that feels real as real can be, while the dream is happening. But, the most remarkable part is that while a dream is happening, another space-time continuum is occurring during the same real-world present moment!

Realizing how a dream world's space-time continuum connects shallower levels of your self-awareness with every dream you dream enables you to comprehend that your self-awareness is a time continuum connecting imagination with a dimension of reality. Such a concept includes the idea that every real-world soul also resonates with a deeper, cosmic self through their shallower degree of self-awareness. Since the real world is similar to another dimension of dreaming, you may consciously care that the real-life universe is a cosmic mind!

Matching the way your dream world's deeper self happens to be you resonating within a multidimensional mind, a real-world deeper self happens to be you resonating within a cosmic mind – the real-life universe. While on a path to get control over deeper subconscious power from the cosmic mind, a deeper thinking ego begins to approach a lucid dream world's level of lucid awareness. Wow! This means you really can consciously believe that every real-life soul is the same self here in the real world, just as every dream soul is the same self in a dream world.

So, how can belief in a real-world cosmic self help you feel some real-life happiness for the long term? Well, by discovering how and why the same self is everyone in the real world, you can consciously care about everyone – your real-time deeper self. This way, a more powerful presence of mind arrives from healthy truth behind a belief that everyone is a shielded degree of the same self. What a wonder! Now you're capable of understanding how, similar to your dream worlds, your real world is also a dimension of existence for the same deeper self – a place where miracles and wonders never cease! A mind that's channelling a dimension of conscious existence is miraculous enough, but the wonder of a space-time continuum feeling perfectly real is the ongoing miracle!

## Aligning With Deeper Self-awareness

I would bet (sportsman's bet) that the greatest wonder of the entire cosmos is a multidimensional mind aligning with an awareness of being somewhere, in some time period, and of really being someone; however, unless linked with a deeper, more powerful real-world presence of mind, this bet won't make much sense to most people. But, by backing away from those conventional standards of thinking, speaking, and behaving, especially the ones lacking deeper imagination, you can follow the unconventional FTBT path. A "Front To Back Thinking" path can align your ego with new awareness that a subconscious mind is the fabric of dream worlds – and the real world.

When, where, why, and with what degree of self-awareness does a lucid dreamer align? Lucid awareness is all about aligning, merging, and fully linking with a multidimensional mind. Deeper FTBT is also all about aligning, merging and linking, except it's an aligned, merged, and connected link with new belief in deeper self-definition. New belief in deeper self-definition can take place because you're capable of comprehending how, comparable to the way a presence of mind is dream reality, a presence of mind is real-life reality.

My lucid dreaming aligns me with deeper self-awareness, makes me understand that the dream's space-time continuum is a field of conscious and subconscious energy, and makes me believe that the entire dream world is a multidimensional mind at play. In the real world, deeper thinking can align you with deeper self-awareness, making you understand how and why the real-world space-time continuum is a field of conscious and subconscious energy, a multidimensional mind at play. Deeper self-awareness boils down to linking up with a more loving game of life because such a link makes your real-world reality automatically (subconsciously) stream forth in a healthy way.

So, how far can you go? Could you possibly align, merge, and fully link with your real-world deeper self? Would you even want to expand your ego into a level of real-world lucid awareness – bringing you into total alignment with a greater self? Could any real person come into a complete alignment with the "One" whose presence of mind is real time and real space, just as a lucid dream character comes into a complete alignment with their greater "One" self – whose presence of mind is the dream world's space time continuum?

During the same instant that a dream is happening, you are all the "Ones" living dream life. Since all real-world self-awareness also connects a present and instantaneous time continuum, a cosmic self is all the "Ones" living real life. That's why a real-life deeper self is also every dream world's deeper self. In other words, all dreams are within a greater dream!

Then again, although lucid awareness makes me consciously aware of being a multidimensional mind at play, my lucid awareness isn't superior (or inferior) to another dream soul's level of self-awareness because concurrently, I am every one of my dream souls. A cosmic real-world deeper self may also be seen in the same light: a cosmic self isn't superior to anyone because a cosmic self is everyone. That's why consciously caring about your deeper self includes caring about all levels of self-awareness. This sort of insight can create new belief in an unconventional FTBT viewpoint. That is, all levels of self-awareness are equal in significance and worthiness because everyone – every "One" – is the same One self.

Same as with dream worlds that aren't lucid (most dreams), there's a critical reason why everyone in the real world is shielded from an all-out alignment, complete connection, and total merge with the cosmic self. Boredom is the reason. Before even considering the possibility of fully waking up and achieving lucid awareness here in the real world, boredom's deeper implications need to be taken into account.

## Strain Due To A Lack Of Stress

Except for the dream soul with lucid awareness, all the consciously aware dream souls in my lucid dream worlds are shielded from any knowledge of my real-world reality. A shielded level of consciousness isn't in alignment with the dreamer. That's why veiled expressions of self-awareness can believe that the dream world is real, and behave accordingly.

I always feel intense relief after new belief arriving with lucid awareness is impressed upon my lucidly aware dream soul. Even so, my lucid awareness can't be egotistical, won't believe in a selfishly greedy outlook that can lead to the formation of prejudiced ideas or opinions about another dream soul. That's because long-lasting lucid awareness brings me a clearer understanding that every dream soul is the same deeper self. All individual dream souls, including those with differing racial, ethnic, or sexually orientated backgrounds add depth to a dream world's space-time continuum. Once again, the dreamer is the creator, and the dreamer's subconscious mind is the creation – all at the same time. That's why a dream world is a self connecting and instantaneous flow of conscious and subconscious energy.

Comprehending the equality of every dream soul's level of self-awareness automatically transforms my outlook. Likewise, while in a deeper thinking, real-world presence of mind, I can comprehend how and why all living organisms – including each and every real person – resemble dream souls that channel the same deeper self. Similar to all the individual levels of shielded self-awareness in a dream world, each and every real-world level of self-awareness may also be viewed as connecting the same deeper self with different outlooks.

During any dimension of reality, a belief in inferior or superior levels of self-awareness clashes with what's really going on! All individuals, regardless of racial, ethnic or sexual background are channelling the same deeper self. As with the nature of lucid awareness during a lucid dream world, there won't be any fearful discrimination or bigotry coming from a healthy, real-world presence of mind. That's because a healthy conscious mind can think deeper!

The deeper I think during my lucid dream fantasies, the closer I get to feeling all-powerful. Deeper thinking lucid awareness has made me understand how and why ultimate subconscious power can eventually end any possibility of surprise. Without the possibility to feel sudden wonder or amazement, especially of something unexpected, my lucid awareness is bound to lead my subconscious mind into a mood of total boredom.

Along with the subconscious creation of an enduring space-time continuum, other escalating superpowers during lucid dream worlds arrive with my ability to make any intention come true. My lucidly aware dream soul can blow down forests, levitate, fly, breathe underwater, pass through solid walls like a ghost, move inanimate objects with just a thought, as well as perform feats of superhuman strength. I can even change into a different person, animal, bird, or anything I want to be. To top off everything, I can even experience my dream soul's death – and ego's out of body experience! Yet, I believe that my greatest subconscious challenge is going to be the creation of new experiences during lucid dream worlds.

Deeper subconscious power comes from the perfectly pure and instantaneous spark of subconscious energy I spoke about earlier, where a huge power surge can happen from feeling zero resistance to boredom. Boredom – the nemesis of ultimate enlightenment – is always on the horizon for ongoing lucid awareness. In other words, ultimate enlightenment and ultimate power equal zero stress which when prolonged, can strain the lucid link.

While considering how complete boredom is an eventual result of ultimate power, you may understand why accomplishing a full alignment with your real-world deeper self is going to instantly feel completely boring. Protection from boredom is what David was talking about during the <u>Golden</u> lucid dream I described in chapter four. While pondering upon that lucid dream, I wondered what David meant with his statement about consciousness being a "protected" version of deeper self-awareness – protected from what? Every dream soul that's shielded from lucid awareness protects the dreamer from eternal boredom!

The answer was there all along, way back in chapter one's <u>Earthy</u> lucid dream. That was the dream in which I discovered how to stay calm during the onset of lucid awareness – I used boredom as a passive correction for my initial giddy and overexcited attitude. This less resistive approach, where I didn't take any steps at all (simply stared at the ground between my feet), eventually brought about a tremendous feeling of boredom. After returning home, I appreciated how complete non-resistance to boredom was no good because I couldn't love the present moment if I was bored out of my mind; therefore, the Lucid Law of Resistance.

For me, lucid dreams continue to channel my interest, excitement, and curiosity about multidimensional existence. I still believe that my lucid dream worlds are miracles from my subconscious mind, but along with greater subconscious power, I can appreciate that eventually, I'll reach a point where I won't feel any delight because there aren't going to be any more surprises.

The number of wonderful new events happening during a lucid dream world won't go on forever because there's going to come a point where there's no getting away from boredom. For example: if you hear a song that you find very beautiful, and listen to it over and over again, you can end up feeling bored with it. Even your favourite movies have limits as to how many times you want to watch and listen to them because eventually, you want to move onto something different.

## The Nemesis Of Ultimate Enlightenment

Just trying to imagine a sensation of perpetual boredom – inevitable after a whole heap of lucid dreaming – helps shed light on an incredible insight involved with a healthier presence of mind. Although complex, this insight can easily be understood by taking a longer look at lucid dreaming.

Eventually, ultimate enlightenment and peak power channelled through lucid awareness are going to make a lucid dream feel tedious. During a very lengthy lucid dream, the lucid dreamer begins to experience repetitive scenarios. After the same ego plays out every conceivable scenario countless times, each possible outcome feels over-rehearsed. Mind-numbing dullness comes from nothing new ever happening, and an ongoing perception of unending boredom sinks in. Perhaps this is why the pinch test during a lucid dream feels like a dull numbness!

Having an immortal and stress-free sensation of consciousness, thanks to boundless superpower, can trap a lucid dreamer into an ongoing state of tedious monotony. Now what to do? Since imagination has no limits, there's a way to relieve a state of perpetual boredom without pinching out: the lucid dreamer can intentionally ignore, forget, and deny lucid awareness by taking a nap from it all. That's because during this nap, the dreamer can experience a dream world without lucid awareness!

Unless lucid, you don't realize you're in a dream world – the dreamer gets ignored, forgotten, denied, and recreated! Along with a shielded mindset, you can experience seemingly new sensations of existence. Boredom – the nemesis of ultimate enlightenment – won't be a problem because fear, anger, and hurt can come back to life. On the upside – harmonious joy, lucid love, and delightful surprise can also come back to life.

Ironically, in order to awaken from perpetual boredom, a new dream world bangs into existence! By imagining to be dream souls who've no idea that they're in a dream world, the dreamer can believe that a different presence of mind is real, without really knowing how or why. That's because an end to the dreamer's eternal monotony arrives with every conscious dream soul's ability to feel surprised!

Unless in a lucid dream world, the dreamer isn't fully awake! Although the same old "song and dance" may repeat, the dreamer connects with seemingly novel experiences through different focus, intention, interpretation, perception, and belief coming from dream souls with shielded levels of conscious self-awareness. Not only that, a dream world's new space-time continuum also exists as an instantaneous now, while during this one present moment, no real space gets taken up. This way, the dreamer can gravitate toward a sensation of novelty for what seems like an eternity, yet, the dream only lasts for an instant. Wow and double wow! Mind boggling? Not really – the equivalent is happening this very moment, in everyone's real-life dimension of reality.

Here in real life, a cosmic self experiences each living soul's awareness of being real. In other words, your deeper self is everywhere because the spirit of life is every living entity – all at the same time. This paradoxical concept happens to be very important to grasp. By viewing dream life from all the different dream souls' points of view at the same time, you're unaware of who, what, or where "you" really are – asleep in another dimension of reality. In fact, you are they!

Throughout any dream fantasy, every dream soul is subconscious energy. Accordingly, every dream soul protects the dreamer from eternal boredom (and death) because dream souls don't fully align, merge, or connect with their own deeper self – unless lucid. A dream soul can have an individual viewpoint and consequent belief system due to the soul's "physical" existence, but deeper down, the living moment for a dream soul is the dreamer's self-awareness. Each dream soul's deeper self is the One dreamer. In this way, the well-worn mind games of a deeper self can become new again!

Consciousness taking place during a regular dream world is very similar to consciousness happening here in the real world. Dream diaries reveal that, for most folks, an individual point of view takes place during a dream world. That is, while you're actually living in a dream world, everything feels real because you don't remember your deeper dimension of existence. That's why a great way to get a more accurate picture of a truer meaning of life is to view the real world as being comparable to another dimension of dreaming. Once again, such an outlook develops from a deeper thinking, real-world presence of mind.

A deeper thinking, real-world presence of mind brings you an ever closer connection with a cosmic self without your aligning, merging, and resonating at the higher harmonic rate capable of achieving ultimate enlightenment. This means that you can continue to experience an existence where everything feels real since you don't remember your cosmic self's deeper dimension of existence. Instead, you can attain a more "perfect" level of enlightenment because healthy trust in having a cosmic self enables you to resist boredom in a lucidly loving way. You can toss fear, anger, and hurt by balancing your subconscious mind with harmonious joy, lucid love, and delightful surprise!

Just as most dream souls don't understand how or why their dimension of reality comes to life, most real-life souls also lack such insight. Plus, conscious energy can impress subconscious energy with a fear of being turned off – in other words, a fear of death. Lucid dreaming brings forth another polished pearl of wisdom that helps a person love the mystery of death because a soul's death protects the spirit of life from boredom.

## Another Step Toward Loving The Mystery Of Death

How can you handle the greater depths of deeper subconscious power without a total transformation of your ego conscious? The short answer is that you can't! Your ego conscious only partially transforms with the deeper power of lucid love.

As you might expect, instead of ignoring, forgetting, and denying who you really are, there happens to be another natural path which avoids monotony in any lucid dream world – coming home! But, who wants to pinch out if you don't have to?

Most of us won't consider pinching out of the real world either; however, an end to your mind game – no matter how well played – eventually arrives after a sufficient aging of your real-world soul. When your human soul dies, your ego can expand with lucid love or if uninformed, you may implode with fear as death's door opens! An informed outlook can bring about belief that while experiencing stress through a shielded ego, ultimate enlightenment can't happen. Since you may comprehend the idea that the same cosmic self is everyone's deeper self, you may also understand why the seven lucid laws apply to every conscious soul. This way, although Lucid Law seems to reward or punish your soul, it's really your own attitude that rewards or punishes – the lucid laws guide and inform.

Conscious and subconscious energy protect deeper self-awareness from the nemesis of ultimate enlightenment – eternal boredom. A deeper thinking mindset reveals why an attitude flowing with lucid love can free you from selfishness and greed without stepping you into a state of total boredom. But, an end to your own guarded mind game, no matter how well you play in dreams or in the real world eventually arrives when your soul stops breathing. Although you may feel lucid love for the long-term, a real-world soul eventually dies of old age. Now the epic question: "What happens to your ego after your real-world soul transforms and death's door opens for you?" The next chapter brings the inevitable answer!

## CHAPTER SIX

# DEATH'S DOOR

There's an age-old saying: "Two things are absolutely certain in life – death and taxes!" If you try to dodge the realism of your tax system, you could suffer from the punishment of a nasty fine and you might even get put in prison. Likewise, if you try to dodge the realism of your own soul's inevitable death, you could also suffer from the punishment of a nasty attitude and you might even get imprisoned in a fearful mood.

Thinking about being taxed to death can feel natural, but thinking about the death of your consciousness can feel unnatural as the nonexistence of time! Yet, you may still try to dodge the inevitability of passing through death's door by making the subject taboo, and for this reason a fear of dying can get impressed upon your soul. As well as facing up to a tax system, facing up to an inevitable transformation of conscious and subconscious energy steps you closer to a truer meaning of death.

The certainty about your own physical body melting back into the earth – along with an uncertainty about the permanence of your ego conscious – can drive a fierce fear, deep down within your soul. This fear revolves around a truer meaning of death! Just trying to imagine the idea of your personality being permanently nonexistent will probably conjure some peculiar and gut wrenching sensations deep down inside of your soul.

A fear of death is one reason why belief in indigenous mythology, or religion can feel so mesmerizing for your subconscious mind. A variety of mythological, or holy ideas taught to people as truthful or correct are about a person's afterlife. Mythological, and holy doctrine teach you to hope (and pray) for your soul to be saved. That's how religion, and indigenous mythology can make people believe that they're inferior to a superior, separate, and judgemental spirit or "God".

The Lucid Boomerang Law explains how and why your thoughts, words, and conduct fly back in rhythm with the subconscious energy you're tapped into. That's why feeling a high hope for a separate soul, or an individual ego to persist for eternity can get you high on hope!

A high hope for your ego to pass through death's door goes against the Lucid Law of Belief's guidance. That's because when the truth behind a belief is unhealthy, you give away your deeper subconscious power. Another person – usually an egotistical bully – may take your subconscious power and use it to make your soul work like a demon! The reason you lose deeper subconscious power is because you're not really loving your present moment.

The Lucid Law of Belief is about making whatever you consciously believe become real as real can be – for your soul. You can get high on conscious belief that your individual ego can live forever due to a subconscious fear of death – until death gets close; then, there's only fear. Deeper thinking offers up a healthier alternative: it's the idea that your ego is the presence of deeper self-awareness. Trusting that your ego is a shielded level of deeper self-awareness can transform all subconscious fear about your passing through death's door because fearful subconscious energy gets tossed when you discover how and why a deeper and immortal self is the real you.

Keeping lucid love's deeper subconscious power flowing within your own soul comes from feeling a trust in everyone's real self being the same One immortal present moment. By understanding why the seven lucid laws are powerful guides that can impress your soul with deeper love for the present moment, you can consciously believe that all seemingly separate levels of self-awareness are the same deeper self. That's why the equality of self-awareness is a natural foundation for Lucid Law.

Once more, the seven lucid laws are: the Lucid Law of Love, Resistance, Tossing Your Burden, Living in the Now, Belief, the Lucid Boomerang Law, and the Lucid Law of Forgiveness. Belief in being linked with a cosmic self gets you some deeper subconscious power to make your attitude work for you instead of against you. In order to make a healthier attitude work for you, you need to feel a love for the path your new ideas and concepts are going to take you on.

When you feel thankful for your life because you love the path you're on, you get lucid love's deeper power to love the present moment that you're experiencing. For example: you may feel thankful for your job because it provides you with a payday, even though you hate your job. But, if you can impress your subconscious mind with a healthier belief in feeling thankful for being present while doing your job, you get lucid love's deeper power to love the present moment that you're experiencing. Jobs are tricky to love because there's often a ladder to climb, and the higher rungs ring with superiority!

As so often happens when a soul is impressed by an ego's belief in worshipping superiority, you may stoop beneath an unhealthy truth behind a belief in your own inferiority, allowing another person to command your world outlook – and mood. Case in point: that a separate and judgemental "God" is superior is a belief that goes against all the lucid laws. Such belief can impress more fear, anger, and hurt upon your subconscious soul because you give away the power to control your own subconscious energy.

A deeper thinking and unconventional view on a superior, separate, and judgemental God helps you grasp how and why the idea of an almighty spirit comes from imagination. Every soul's self-awareness is the real essence of indigenous mythology as well as holy doctrine, yet, the real essence of self-awareness is the present moment. That's why a deeper thinking person can go along with the idea that the real spirit of life is an all-time presence of self-awareness. This way, the present moment may be thought of as being a cosmic presence for all of eternity!

Once more, there's a notable drawback with belief that you're inferior to a superior, separate, and judgemental God – you give away your deeper subconscious power. A cosmic self is always with you, here and now, no matter who or where you are. Instead of hoping and praying for your ego to experience a happy afterlife, a trust in your deeper self being immortal gets you some deeper subconscious power to love a greater presence of mind. That's because this greater presence of mind is the present moment.

Firstly, you have scientific proof of a deeper self – your own dream worlds! Secondly, a high hope to personally pass through death's door can be a slippery slope into an age-old nightmare. If you allow yourself to be bullied, owing to the devious idea of your personality passing through death's door, you aren't giving love to the present moment. If you spend your life suffering, while waiting for some beautiful and magical place in an afterlife, you may never learn to love, cherish, and connect with the one perfectly present moment that you're in!

## A Fear Of Death

Another reason why some people think that their ego might outlive bodily death comes from belief in paranormal demons and angels. I won't deny the possibility of ghostly spirits existing since I too have experienced some very strange real-world encounters with the supernatural.

A ghost is usually considered to be the spiritual energy of someone's consciousness – a conscious attitude that remains after bodily death. Some people believe that the spiritual presence of somebody who has died can appear as a shadowy form or cause sounds, the movement of objects, or a frightening atmosphere in a place. After a person's soul stops breathing, their ego may have an out of body experience (OBE) and stay aware of what's going on. Such an afterlife can only be temporary unless there's a compatible energy source available to sustain the disembodied presence of an ego, and this is one reason why ghostly spirits come into contact with the living – to get energy from another subconscious soul by helping to satisfy that soul's hunger.

At first, this view of a food chain may feel disagreeable, but it's really just a different way to look at how and why conscious and subconscious energy transform. By merging with your subconscious mind, a ghostly spirit of conscious energy can continue to feel alive! Although a mean-spirited ghost may appear to have an unhealthy attitude, this is really all about energy transforming. Real-life people can have unhealthy attitudes that are hauntingly energetic, and such nasty minded thinking gets fed from fearful, angry, and hurtful subconscious energy. Then again, a person can have a heavenly attitude. A heavenly attitude gets fed from lucidly loving, harmoniously joyful, and delightfully surprising states of subconscious energy.

Another reason for this view of disturbing, and heavenly energy being the subconscious mind's food for channelling a conscious attitude is that such a concept can make you ask more questions about your own self-definition. I've had to consciously ask: "Is my conscious energy egotistical? Am I trying to transform an unhealthy attitude into a healthy one?" My answer: "Yes." I had to face this monstrous level of self-definition because I needed to pass through it! A healthier attitude gets powered by a lucidly loving outlook; however, an egotistical outlook still provides relief from eternal boredom, even though it may make consciousness short-lived!

## The Thunderbird Lucid Dream

A remarkable event relating to death's door occurred during one of those earlier, deeper thinking lucid dreams – when I was learning to remain calm in order to avoid returning home prematurely. At the beginning of this lucid dream world, I knelt in a moonlit meadow. Far from civilization and deep in raw nature, the dimly lit place was alive with early evening sounds. Along with a hooting owl, some crickets and frogs filled the air with a continuous chirring and croaking which created a musical atmosphere.

After what seemed like a long measure of the magical moment, I moved my attention from the small patch of warm earth where I was kneeling, zoomed in on the sudden silence right next to me. A frolicking frog had suddenly stopped croaking – the strange looking little beast was dead. My sorrow transformed into delightful surprise as I became transfixed by a marble sized bubble which rose slowly into the twilight! Having departed from the frog's body, the little droplet contained a rainbow of radiant energy; I watched it drift up into the soft sky.

All at once, an enormous and translucent birdlike creature appeared overhead. About the size of a light, two-seat airplane and outlined by vast wings spread wide, the shimmering predator flew toward the sparkling little droplet of energy. After one sharp snap of the alien bird's immense beak, the frog's globe of radiance was gone! The creature abruptly turned a greenish hue while circling the meadow, and the name "Thunderbird" echoed in my mind. Just before this lucid dream ended, I brought my stunned attention back down to the ground where dozens of tiny coloured orbs emanated from a swampy area in front of me – mosquitoes and flies were dying.

The next morning, after reading through my dream diary, I chewed on the thought of hungry Thunderbirds eating conscious and subconscious energy. Dreaming about bubbles of energy rising from dying souls was a way for me to understand that conscious and subconscious energy could boil out of a soul after the soul died. I thought about how the energy bubble ascending from a person's dead body might be large, complex, and very tasty relative to that of a frog or fly! This idea made me question how – after my soul died – could I save my departing orb of energy from being gobbled up by a hungry Thunderbird, or by some other beast even higher up on the cosmic food chain? The thought of a paranormal predator feeding on a soul's departing droplet of energy became a huge concern for me, and I wondered if such incidents could account for our legendary tales of bitter demons – and sweet angels.

My belief about the meaning of death has transformed over the decades. A more flexible viewpoint on this really important subject has been evolving with my healthier Front To Back Thinking (FTBT). For one thing, the idea that energy can boil out of a dying soul explains why there's more to every creature's death than instant oblivion. Death is food for further thought!

At this point, sharing some concerns about everyone eventually departing from their real-world soul helps bring home a deeper thinking mindset. Discussing death from a deeper FTBT point of view enables peace of mind with respect to a truer meaning of death.

In my late forties and throughout my fifties, I worked at the Royal Jubilee Hospital power plant in Victoria, British Columbia, (Canada). While working as a certified power engineer in the hospital's power plant, I was responsible for the HVAC equipment – heating, ventilation and air-conditioning – as well as hot and cold potable water systems, emergency generators, diesel, nitrogen and oxygen supply systems, to name but a few! With seventeen operating rooms and three floors of specialized clinics, along with dozens of large buildings spread over several acres, the Royal Jubilee is the biggest hospital on Vancouver Island. For over ten years, I worked throughout the hospital and became skilled at interacting with lots of patients – some close to death! Many of these folks had interesting beliefs about a deeper meaning of death. Occasionally, we would get into brief conversations about dreaming.

Patients who appeared to be calm and sensible would usually speak happily about healthy dream worlds where joy flourished and dream life went fairly smoothly; however, these types of attitudes were few and far between. The vast majority of people who spoke with me weren't happy, but whether optimistic or glum, almost everyone was interested in talking about their dream worlds!

Those more upbeat folks who could once see, but had become blind explained to me that while dreaming, they had picture perfect twenty/twenty vision! As well, happier minded crippled people – the one's who appeared to be coping with their stark and sterile hospital environment – spoke about walking and running without pain while in their dream worlds. And, many of the more friendly deaf people told me that while dreaming, they could hear perfectly well without any hearing aids. Here was some real evidence that patients who experienced healthy levels of self-awareness in their dream worlds had happier real-world outlooks. Strangely enough, not one person out of the hundreds that I spoke with ever reported a realization of being in a dream world while the dream was happening, or had ever even heard of lucid dreaming.

These folks helped me understand how a healthier truth behind the real meaning of life is really about why a deeper and greater dreamer has been ignored, forgotten, and denied. A healthy dream is about more than just relieving the presence of ultimate enlightenment's perpetual boredom, it's about relieving boredom in ways that feel good.

Remarkably, nurses insisted upon opening the nearest window, immediately, after a patient's death; I was always told that time was of the essence and to make sure the maintenance workers kept the old hospice wing's working windows in good working order! That's because some sort of presence would depart after a person's body died.

For those people who are heartbroken, traumatized, lonely, depressed, knocking on death's door, or maybe even knocking on heaven's door, and are also seeking a point to life, stepping into a healthier presence of mind brings a real answer. The deepest and greatest answer to what life is really all about turns out to be surprisingly straightforward: it's all about channelling a different level of self-awareness in order to toss perpetual boredom.

A dream world is a presence of mind imagining and living a dimension of existence during a self connecting moment in order to realize differing depths of self-awareness. The real world is also a presence of mind imagining and living a dimension of existence during a self-connecting moment in order to realize differing depths of self-awareness.

During a dream world's present moment, a dream character can believe that their real self is a separate expression of self-awareness. Expressed with parallel power, real-world people also seem to believe that their real self is a separate expression of self-awareness. But, by going in the reverse direction, a more practical way to discover the true meaning of life arrives from understanding why your real self is actually the opposite of being separate because deeper self-awareness is "One" and all.

If you choose to look, you can notice how everyone experiences their real-world reality concurrently. Again, getting straight to the point (from a deeper thinking viewpoint), we're all equal in so far as self-awareness goes because every living soul channels the same deeper self. Belief in every soul's deeper self being the same dreamer can also channel lucid love into life!

Playing a cosmic game of life gives you a precious sensation of being an individual person who feels real. Animals, birds, fish, insects, plants, and absolutely everything else living within every space-time continuum – including paranormal entities – also have self-awareness. Having a shielded and protected level of self-awareness that resists boredom (and death's door) is the real point to a cosmic self playing the game of life.

## An Alert!

There's a dangerous, razor-sharp risk involved with believing that the real world is a cosmic dimension of dreaming. Because a cosmic self happens to be immortal, there's an audacious and provocative possibility that nothing really matters; however, understanding Lucid Law alerts you about such risky thinking.

The lucid laws are powerful pointers helping to step you in a healthy direction because for one thing, everything really does matter! I'll always cherish my <u>Soul Saving</u> lucid dream, the lucid dream that taught me how to return home without having to physically pinch out. I remember feeling a razor-sharp sorrow before returning home from the merciful and lifesaving lucid dream world that I described near the end of chapter one. That was the lucid dream during which I gained incredible subconscious power while loving the present moment, then accidentally blew down the beautiful forest. Before I returned home, I felt a huge loss after the devastating way in which my loving link with life in the forest was severed. That's because all those shielded and unique dream souls were "killed". After returning home, I thought: "Since everything was a dream, no one was actually killed – it was a deeper presence of mind that got transformed."

If you lose the lovely link with your present moment, the loss can shock your own subconscious soul, and you may feel heartbroken. But, if you can step into a deeper thinking mindset – as I'll explain in the upcoming chapters – and connect with greater reasoning for loving your present moment, you can toss overwhelming shock coming from personal disasters!

A healthy step onward, from having to let go of a partner, family member, friend, or a pet – due to their soul's death – can take place with your immersion into deeper subconscious power. This sort of power comes from conscious belief in forgiveness, which I'll also explain in more detail in the following chapters. Showing sympathy for the suffering of all souls goes along with the Lucid Law of Forgiveness where, for example, you can forgive cutting thoughts, words, and deeds delivered by egotistical points of view because compassion connects you with deeper subconscious power – the power to transform an unhealthy outlook. This way, when you know how to heal your own slashed heart, you're safe to love your own present moment of self-awareness once again!

Although a dream world is only an illusion, all the dream souls' points of view, emotions, and experiences feel real for the dreamer. In order to avoid falling into the trap of believing that nothing really matters because everything physical is really subconscious energy, you need only appreciate the idea that all levels of self-awareness are the same spirit of life. That's why everything really does matter! This is a matter for serious thought because the cosmic self is a creator and consumer of emotional energy, the original giver and taker, the real One who is the life force feeding a cosmic food chain!

Getting back to the concept of your real world being just like a dream world, why would you want to believe that a greater dreamer has denied you memory of who you really are? Because this way, you can comprehend why you're always connected with a deeper and greater self. You can gain some real courage to trust that your real self is immortal! Deducing this realization of immortality – through the study of your dream worlds – can bring you some deeper subconscious power to believe in a healthy truth behind the meaning of life. For one thing, you can free yourself from any fear of death.

For sure you want to live, but the thought of your soul's death needn't paralyze you with fear. You can feel a heavenly mood when you believe that a deeper and "greater" self's subconscious mind is the fabric for a cosmic dimension of existence. Once more, thanks to the miracle of your shielded and protected viewpoint, you help abolish eternal boredom for a greater presence of mind – a "Great One Dreamer".

The concept of a Great One Dreamer being food for thought can get you some deeper and healthier subconscious power to channel lucid love into your present moment. Although all levels of self-awareness in any dream world equal the dream world's deeper self, unless lucid, a dream character is unaware that their deeper presence of mind is multidimensional. Then again, a lucidly aware presence of mind understands why the dream world's present moment is self-aware. The identical principle may be applied here in the real world where all levels of self-awareness equal a real-world deeper self.

An ego can realize a healthier outlook through their soul's healthy mood, or realize a disturbing outlook through their soul's unhealthy mood; however, one way or another, your soul is going to eventually melt back into the Earth, and you're going to pass through death's door. So, what really happens when you die? An accurate answer to this question can become quite clear when analyzed from a deeper thinking viewpoint because your real-life self (the real you) cannot perish! Physical bodies melt back into the earth to enrich the fabric of a greater subconscious soul, and an ego also transforms in order to enrich a deeper and greater presence of mind.

Realization that your real self is a Great One Dreamer can impress your own soul with belief that the essence of your life is immortal. This way, you might save your departing orb of self-awareness from being gobbled up by a beastly Thunderbird, or by some other brute even higher up on the cosmic food chain!

Your ego is going to transform as you awaken from a real-world dimension of reality. The subconscious moods you've felt within your own soul give direction to the way your transformation flows onward. That's because your soul's deeper moods add a certain flavour to your ego's attitude.

A deeper meaning of death is all about subconscious hunger for the flavour of presence that departs from a soul. That's how and why an unhealthy ego feeds fear, anger, and hurt into the present moment. Then again, a healthy ego can feed harmonious joy, lucid love, and delightful surprise into the present moment!

## Re-Birth

Your present, real-world dimension of existence may appear to be your only real reality, and your thoughts on death may be filled with fear. Applying to birth as well as death, another age-old adage is that history repeats. More precisely, instead of exact history actually occurring again, the way in which your attitude harmonizes with your subconscious soul brings recurring moods to match.

On one hand, human beings are capable of channelling conscious self-awareness through their more evolved souls. On the other hand, egotistical fervour doesn't recognize a deeper truth behind the meaning of life. Today, an enormous number of people appear to believe that superior self-awareness feels real. To top it off, many folks also seem to believe in the idea that some sort of a spiritual being is an all-time, superior entity. Again and again, human history repeats with such conscious belief manifesting disturbing moods. Fear, anger, and hurt boil out of such egotistical fervour!

People's subconscious minds hear business, political, and religious leaders informing citizens from all walks of life that God is a separate and omnipotent judge! Along with this measure of direction, there's always the superior and the inferior, whereas within a lucidly loving presence of mind, there's equality with everyone ("every One").

In spite of egotism, a rigid belief in any superior level of self-awareness ensures a lively resistance to boredom in the real world and in dream worlds! There're big and small battles, wars, and lots of fighting taking place all over the planet. Such devout conflicts testify to the mayhem coming from a hunger for superiority. Not only that, the big question about why a greater dreaming mind would allow so much pain and suffering to take place can be answered – you're the "One" channelling fear, anger, and hurt! You create your own painful and unhappy space-time continuum by channelling an unhealthy attitude.

The same way every dream soul channels life from a greater subconscious mind, every real-world soul also channels life from a greater subconscious mind. As far as death goes, all dream souls seem to suddenly disappear after your dream ends; however, all the shielded levels of self-awareness add depth to your own mind as you awaken from sleep.

After a real person dies, the person's shielded level of self-awareness also seems to suddenly disappear. Once again, every soul's presence of mind transforms by way of deeper subconscious power. A powerful poem written by Mary Frye may help you grasp this lucid glimpse of life and death:

> Do not stand at my grave and weep;
> I am not there. I do not sleep.
> I am a thousand winds that blow.
> I am the diamond glints on snow.
> I am the sunlight ripened grain;
> I am the gentle autumn rain.
> When you awaken in the morning hush,
> I am the swift uplifting rush,
> Of quiet birds in circled flight,
> I am the soft stars that shine at night.
> Do not stand at my grave and cry;
> I am not there. I did not die!
>
> Mary Frye, <u>Do Not Stand at My Grave and Weep</u>

I interpret the poem to be about a person's ego transforming – after their soul's death. Although your own subconscious soul is going to transform by melting back into the earth, or maybe first becoming dust in the wind, your ego can appear to vanish by boiling off and evaporating. Even with lucid love providing meaningfulness for what's going on around you, you'll probably still resist the inevitability of an ending for your own brain, heart, body and soul because your ego wants to live the dream! That's why the Lucid Law of Resistance is also about resisting a total merge with the cosmic self.

By resisting your own merge with ultimate enlightenment, you protect yourself from total boredom. This means ultimate enlightenment won't take place after your real soul's death since ultimate boredom strains an ego's link with lucid awareness; however, when your bodily soul does die, your lucidly loving level of conscious energy can feed a greater subconscious mind with some healthy food for thought!

A deeper FTBT outlook lights up the idea that everyone's sensation of "here and now" is a combination of subconscious and conscious energy. Health may be viewed as an imaginative thought, a place where there's balance to conscious and subconscious energy. During dream worlds as well as in the real world, when any level of self-awareness passes through death's door, that level of self-awareness transforms their present moment with fresh food for thought.

A fear of death is what makes the illusion of dying seem so daunting! During dream worlds and in the real world, your deeper self serves up living entities who don't perceive that they're essentially imaginative states of subconscious energy, and the novelty of a physical dimension of existence can feel real; nevertheless, from a balanced mind, you can trust that similar to a dream world's deeper self, a real-world deeper self is also immortal. That's why you may toss the burden of fearing death's door!

After any soul's bodily death, their real self persists in a self connecting present moment. Any soul's fatality in the real world can be seen to parallel a dream soul's demise in so far as a soul's level of self-awareness transforms into a different presence of mind. For example: plenty of people are killed instantly in car accidents, wars, family disputes, extreme weather, and so on… and their egos seem to suddenly vanish into thin air!

Another significant parallel between a real-world ego and a dream world ego is that just as a dream soul's awareness of the dream world suddenly vanishes when that dream soul dies, the real world is also going to seem to suddenly vanish when your real-world soul dies. Plus, the real world really does disappear from your conscious mind every night when you go to sleep. Yet, you may still ask: "What will become of my ego after I actually die?

Understanding how dream worlds are valid dimensions of reality allows you to free your ego from many sinister traps associated with egotism, your space-time continuum measurements, and death's door. That's because when you understand where your ego comes from, you can realize an inevitable return to completion. But, where does your deeper, greater, and complete self – the cosmic self – come from? Without transcending all the way into a state of complete boredom, having lucid awareness during a lucid dream world reveals the real answer! This answer arrives before the end of this chapter! The first clue is that a brain doesn't create self-awareness.

A soul's type of brain, hormones due to gender, ancestry, plus category of environment work to channel subconscious energy into consciousness. In other words, if you were to reach a level of real-life lucid awareness, your ego would be blown away and replaced with a new identity – an uncaring and all-time bored One! That's why a shallower level of self-awareness turns out to be most perfect since you can continue to resist boredom, and live like a livewire!

## Reincarnation

Lots of people believe that reincarnation is a cyclic return of the same ego. But, is a belief in the rebirth of your own ego conscious accurate? And, how hard is it to change an inaccurate belief? For many people, a bad tempered mood results from another person trying to change their firm and considered opinion!

In a safe way, a way that's capable of carrying you into a good tempered mood, deeper insight into reincarnation helps clear any misconception about an ego's rebirth. For example: hypnosis enables a person to focus calmly while in a physically and mentally peaceful state, a place where deeper memory can wake up. There happens to be a huge opportunity for you to go way back in your subconscious mind's deeper memory, before your soul was even born!

We've got many explanations for someone thinking of and describing earlier lifetimes while under hypnosis. Believing that an individual's ego can get reborn is what reincarnation is all about. There're many documented cases of people speaking foreign languages while regressed into a past life, as well as these same people describing places that really existed – along with events that actually happened! Hypnosis seems to confirm the concept of the same ego having lived past lives. You can go on the internet and search "past lives through hypnosis" to see numerous documented cases that try to prove what appears to be the rebirth of the same ego – reincarnation.

My FTBT (and scientific) explanation of how reincarnation works can return deeper insight: subconscious memories from ancestors are passed down through a gene pool via DNA. DNA stands for Deoxyribonucleic Acid, which is a molecule encoding genetic instructions used in the development and functioning of all known living organisms. When a person's body (or any soul) gets born, cellular memory appears. Your DNA's genetic instructions are super dense particles of subconscious energy (subconscious memories) being passed down through your gene pool. And, I'm sure you've heard that great joke about what one DNA molecule asked another DNA molecule: "Do these genes make me look fat?

Thanks to DNA, a human baby bares the essence of life – self-awareness – from each parents' soul, which makes sense because a baby's soul comes from a man and a woman, after each parent bares their own soul! This way, every human baby gets imprinted with it's mother's and father's cellular memories. Not only that, parents carry an impression from their mother and father's souls, and back it goes, just like Front To Back Thinking!

Life keeps flowing onward due to each newborn soul being encoded with the DNA of ancestors. That's why every soul can grow with new complexity. For instance: human souls have an inherent ability to learn an ancestral language, and some can easily learn how to read and write since skills also get passed down through the gene pool. An ancestor's skill – such as making music – may return as a talent, and talents can evolve.

Accessing memory from a period before your soul was born is possible because up to a certain point, your DNA carries memory impressed by ancestors. The cut-off point is during birth. Through hypnosis, you may remember some sensation of your mother's beliefs up until the point where she gave birth, and also recall your father's beliefs up to about nine months before your soul was born. Same from your mother and father's parents, and their parents' parents, and so on. Remembering and describing earlier lifetimes while under hypnosis is really linked with beliefs from ancestors!

Aligning your own ego with a past life – through hypnotic regression – lights up wondrous memory from your own subconscious mind and rationalizes why every level of individual self-awareness has lived past lives! All you need do is calm your soulful mood into a trance state in order to align your ego with deeper subconscious memory, the sort of memory that enables your own shielded level of self-awareness to regress!

After returning to your present branch of ego conscious, your belief system can evolve. Once again, more steps onward – once you're going in a lucidly loving direction – creates a natural flow toward your achieving "perfect" enlightenment. That's why linking with a lucidly loving presence of mind is easy. Even a slow pace can keep you on track toward your own peace of mind because you're advancing. Your subconscious mind's deeper power becomes far easier to control if you can view your own birth as the rebirth of a cosmic self.

## Original Human Consciousness

The original birth of human consciousness has a good scientific explanation. There's speculation that the beginning of the physical universe (and time) arrived with an explosion of energy, as has been suggested by the popular scientific Big Bang theory. This scientific theory is also about an alignment of natural ingredients that continue to channel primordial levels of subconscious self-awareness.

Here on planet Earth, natural elements coalesce into basic subconscious cellular patterns that channel life as we know it. And, cellular patterns continue to provide the building blocks for the present moment to evolve through what you may now realize is a means for self-awareness to connect with consciousness – subconscious energy in the form of a physical soul.

The rebirth of your ego (reincarnation) also has a scientific explanation – DNA. A human ego is the presence of cosmic energy because an ego is a shielded level of an immortal time continuum. In this case, I've used the word "shielded" to signify how consciousness arrives in a way that's easily described by the idea of the Lucid Boomerang Law: subconscious memory has an effect on conscious energy. This means that the quality of your current life is determined by your thoughts, words, behaviour, and by your ancestor's thoughts, words, and behaviour!

A healthy outlook is able to ground your present level of self-awareness by helping you love the idea of having a guarded connection with a cosmic self – a protected link with a greater cosmic presence of space and time. This way, although deeper thinking is still in a state of veiled self-awareness (not fully awake), such thinking enables you to trust that your cosmic self is a universal dimension of time and space. Such trust (not hope) allows you to toss antagonized and resentful attitudes! The reason you can toss burdening egotistical attitudes is because healthier thinking makes you appreciate why your presence is the expression of an immortal and universal self!

While in human form, your ego grants you a choice in how you interpret and perceive your existence, and knowing this can provide some courage for you to trust that you're much more than just an egotistical fool! You're capable of uniting with a belief in your deeper and greater self being everybody's deeper and greater self, and your ego can impress your soul from a more compassionate point of view.

Balancing deeper thinking with lucid love guarantees you protection from perpetual boredom, also guaranteeing a healthier ego conscious. By realizing the significance of a more accurate view on reincarnation, as well as how and why cellular memories are a functioning part of a greater subconscious mind, you may also appreciate why some of the most unhealthy impressions on a soul are the ones resulting from trauma!

Bringing conscious and subconscious awareness into balance enables you to toss traumatized subconscious energy – the bad sort of subconscious memory that can continue to energize unhealthy attitudes. Case in point: if an ancestor was brutally heart-broken, you could be burdened by their original stress disorder. Quite possibly, an ancestor's soul may have survived a traumatic event before contributing to the creation of a family. War veterans are typical examples: perhaps a great grandfather suffered severely due to the death of beloved comrades in combat, and some unhealthy subconscious memory came down through your gene pool. If no subsequent relative in your lineage was able to release the frozen terror from the initial traumatizing event, you're going to continue feeling the hurt deep down inside of your soul.

Every so often, you may feel disturbing sensations of shock from the mood of a subconscious memory being fed back to life by your subconscious mind. Turning to the Lucid Law of Forgiveness for help – as I'll explain further in the following chapters – enables you to toss these types of subconscious stress disorders.

Even if your subconscious memory is healthy, a perception of life as being boring won't last long while living in the real world! Appropriate to the regular stress of real-life self-awareness, there's always going to be some novelty thanks to your resistive and live – like a live-wire – ego.

Dream diaries prove subconscious energy makes dream worlds feel real and that the dreaming mind is incredibly important for health. Also, the question about where the cosmic self comes from can finally be answered: all levels of self-awareness loop full circle to create the presence of time! This way, death's door is the pathway to your own rebirth. Living in an instantaneous "here and now" dimension of existence is real-life resistance to death's perpetual boredom. That's why the real question is: where does self-awareness come from? A level of self-awareness comes from a soul's taste for life!

The cosmic mind is just like a "Great One Dreamer", One who sleeps with purpose. An ego conscious helps save the cosmic mind from perpetual boredom because an ego guards their soul from a full on merge with an all-time deeper and greater self. Being similar to a dimension of dream reality, the physical universe is another side to the cosmic mind – the subconscious side. This means that the universe is a place where incredibly, memories and feelings help shape the patterns channelling subconscious energy into conscious energy. Stirring up lucid love, you can help shape the real world into a healthier pattern of conscious existence!

Similar to Dreamtime, real time is conscious and subconscious energy. A world famous German-born theoretical physicist – Albert Einstein (1879-1955) said that "Energy can be neither created nor destroyed." But, you may still ask where energy originally came from. It's the same thing as asking where self-awareness originally came from. All energy is a state of mind that comes from resistance to boredom, and boredom comes from pure subconscious power accompanying ultimate enlightenment! That's why the more enlightened you become, the more dreamlike your reality appears to be and by the same token, the less enlightened you are, the more real you feel. While in a level of "perfect" enlightenment, even an illusion can feel really good!

For the sake of brevity, an acronym for the name "Great One Dreamer" can be used... GOD. The cosmic mind may also be referred to as "GOD" because deeper Front To Back Thinking proves how and why an unconventional concept of a Great One Dreamer being everybody's deeper self is heavenly food for thought!

# CHAPTER SEVEN

# YOU'RE NOT SUPERIOR TO ANYONE; NO WAY!

Many a time, I've come home from a lucid dream world that seemed to last a lifetime! After writing in my dream diary, I'd eventually ask myself: "What day is it?" Then I'd wonder what month I was in, and after calmly realizing that I'd even forgotten what year I was in, I'd always feel thankful for today – my favourite day!

Not everyone feels that "today" is their favourite day. Some people have formidable levels of unbalanced conscious and subconscious energy to cope with. In the real world as well as in dream worlds there may be bullying sorts of souls who hunger for a belief in superiority, and you might even have your own spasms of egocentricity to contend with.

Formidable levels of unbalanced conscious and subconscious energy can bring about unhealthy moods; people can get so deranged as to declare that all of existence is a plane of suffering. Ironically, feeling these types of unhealthy moods offers a window of opportunity to channel a lucidly loving presence of mind because knowing how you don't want to feel can remind you about how you do want to feel.

Giving lucid love brings about healthier subconscious energy from within your own mind, body, heart and soul, and from the cosmic mind – the present space-time continuum. That's because your own soul and the cosmic soul get impressed by your ego's conscious belief in loving the present moment. Plus, you can show respect for the presence of all souls when you're able to calmly realize that the same deeper self is everyone.

Because a lucidly aware dream soul is channelling the dreamer's ego conscious, a lucid dream only ever has one lucidly aware presence of mind taking place at a time. While linked with lucid awareness, the dreamer can direct the lucid dream world in such a heavenly way that inevitably, all hardship may be overcome; then, there's constant bliss.

Constant bliss can get mind numbingly boring because there's a cold and broken hallelujah going along with a lack of any sort of surprise. Total control over subconscious power strains lucid awareness since along with total control, there's no being caught unawares. Without any possibility for delightful surprise, ultimate power eventually fails to feel good. In order to return from this sort of failure, a step back into a shallower level of self-awareness is a healthier step onward!

Thankfully, here in the real world, an ego saves One from ultimate enlightenment, ultimate power, and ultimate boredom. That's because the whole point of channelling an ego conscious is to step the cosmic self into a healthier level of enlightenment.

Although egotism is automatically (subconsciously) tossed by a healthy level of enlightenment, suddenly being faced with another person's egotistical outlook can feel challenging! That's why conscious belief in compassion and respect – from a lucidly loving point of view – frames the kind of real-world attitude best suited to handle such an aggressive surprise.

## **Aggressive Surprise**

Suddenly facing an aggressive workplace, home, schoolyard, or any brand of egotistical bully can feel surprisingly unpleasant, given that you may believe there's no way to escape! But, you're capable of showing respect and compassion for all levels of self-awareness by reminding yourself about guidance from Lucid Law. A deeper interpretation of a few relevant lucid laws helps make clear how an intention to love the present moment can help you easily survive a hostile, or violent surprise.

You might agree with the idea that bullying comes from a selfishly greedy outlook. An egotistical outlook proves that superior self-awareness is believable! Belief in having a superior level of self-awareness is another fine example of why subconscious fear can return like a boomerang, bringing unhappiness in the long run. That's because such conscious belief has a subconscious counterpart – fear of being inferior. In a harsh way, an egotistical outlook serves to reveal the plight of ignoring deeper understanding pouring from the Lucid Boomerang Law.

A person who fears a bully may realize a nightmarish outlook and typically – blames the bully! Rational and clear, FTBT helps make you more aware of what's really going on. When you feel a genuine trust in your deeper self being everyone's deeper self, the empowerment can mellow your own soul's displeasure, and your outlook can change direction.

Even if surrounded by an entire group of bullies, lucidly loving energy helps calm tense situations since you're consciously caring about every One. Loving the present moment that you're experiencing transforms fearful subconscious energy into a calmer state. When your own mood calms down, you may once again appreciate that we're all the same deeper self. This way, you can show sympathy for the suffering that accompanies an egotistical point of view, often with a desire to help. There's no need to fear, blame, or resist with resentment if you can love sharing the present moment with another perception of yourself because just like a boomerang, lucid love loops back!

Conscious belief in having a loving connection with your deeper and greater One self impresses your own subconscious mind with more than enough power to toss all fear of any aggressive attitude. Trusting that your own deeper self is also everybody's deeper self guides you into believing in the Lucid Law of Love, and helps explain why one person's lucidly loving outlook can calm another person's unhealthy mood. From a lucidly loving outlook, you're able to bring about the kind of communication capable of creating healthier moods. Healthier moods begin with your own lucidly loving attitude sharing a real respect for all the lucid laws, which once again are: the Lucid Law of Love, Resistance, Tossing Your Burden, Living in the Now, Belief, the Lucid Boomerang Law, and the Lucid Law of Forgiveness.

If you only remember one Lucid Law, let it be the deepest one – the Lucid Law of Love. A lucidly loving presence of mind makes more lucid love fly back at you because sharing a love for living in the present moment with another person – even if they're in an egotistical mindset – also shares deeper love for yourself. Lucid love returns automatically, thanks to the connection between your own subconscious soul and your cosmic soul.

## Happy Life

If you choose to feel thankful for all those "demanding" souls with egotistical attitudes, owing to their show of selfish pride reminding you about how you don't want to feel, you can take a different path than that of an egotist. Wanting to transform your own selfish and greedy attitude brings you a healthy reason to look more wholeheartedly at all seven lucid laws. That's because transforming an unhealthy attitude is easy if you can love the idea of Lucid Law.

Loving new ideas and concepts arriving with a deeper understanding of Lucid Law transforms an egotistical outlook. Belief in everyone being connected with the same multidimensional mind is infinitely greater and far more powerful than belief in everyone being disconnected because belief in connection enables a person to channel lucid love. This way, lucid love helps you to outlive another person's egotistical folly. For instance: while you're pouring out a love for the presence of a real-life moment, with no strings attached, even a bully can eventually smile back at you!

Believing that a Great One Dreamer (GOD) is you can impress your soul with a good mood, and you can face formidable levels of conscious and subconscious energy, without feeling fear. An intention behind the idea of your deeper self being a Great One Dreamer is to toss boredom by way of healthy moods that can survive for the long-term. With a lucidly loving attitude in place, you feed your mind with healthy truth behind belief in self-respect and compassion instead of so much unhealthy truth behind belief in selfishness and greed!

You may free yourself from belief in superiority – which also makes a fear of inferiority feel real – because freedom comes from the fairness of lucid love. Lucid love is based on the equality of all self-awareness. When you're free from believing in superior and inferior levels of self-awareness, your selfish and greedy attitudes transform!

If you judge a person to be primitive because you believe that their attitude is bossy and ignorant, then instead of merely acknowledging another example of your deeper self's suffering, you can fear what you believe to be horribly ugly – bullying! Unless you want to encourage bullying, despite the fact that it's likely to have a damaging effect on your own subconscious mind, you might want to think about egotism from front to back.

A belief in superior and inferior levels of self-awareness is going to create the opposite of an intention to stop a bully's bull! Through a lucidly loving attitude, you can chant loudly, "You're NOT superior to anyone; NO way!" This chant facilitates the transformation of consciousness – your consciousness. Such a loud mantra tosses your anger. Tossing an angry emotional response makes way for a healthy path into a lucidly loving outlook.

By understanding the deeper direction of lucid love, and believing in the equality of self-awareness, you can keep stepping onward, into the life that you want to live. Faith in the fairness of lucid love shows why you don't need to fear what might happen when you chant the mantra, "You're NOT superior to anyone; NO way!" That's because a subconscious connection automatically flies back at you – you're NOT inferior; NO way!

More and more bullying attitudes can come to life if you pander to another's unhealthy subconscious mood because your fear of an "inferior" thug can definitely cause you to be duped and fleeced by your own ignorance! Within a lucidly loving mindset, there's no fearful hate, fierce anger, or resentment while chanting: "You're NOT superior to anyone; NO way!", to any aggressive person who's trying to intimidate you. When you believe in the equality of another person's level of self-awareness, your lucid love shines through.

Most folks are likely to shelter some shady attitudes. Having an ego means bad attitudes are always around, even though you may want to step into a lucidly loving outlook. Many shadowy and fearful attitudes exist for a conscious outlook because being able to glimpse into the shadows is one way to stay free from complete boredom!

Shady attitudes may demand that a "superior" Samaritan save "inferior" and brutish thugs from starving to death. For example: if a wealthy person wants to help feed drug addicted street people, a lucidly loving outlook makes clear that wealthy individuals don't have superior levels of self-awareness. Knowing that everyone's ego is equal in significance and worthiness protects you from idolizing another soul.

Raising whatever you believe are profound types of questions, while keeping in mind that your real-world reality happens to parallel a dimension of dream reality, you need only wait for subconscious energy to create solutions, automatically. You don't need to try to solve so many complications from your ego's point of view – you may toss that beastly burden! A happy mood becomes automatic when a belief in lucid love becomes subconscious!

## A Paradox of Self-awareness

Shielded levels of self-awareness are the real point of life. Questioning, testing, acknowledging, and eventually believing that your real world is similar to another miraculous dimension of dreaming can reveal why an instantaneous Great One Dreamer (GOD) gets dreamt into existence! Since this GOD is in fact wholly and one hundred percent "you", your ego makes for a fresh breath of shallower, shielded self-awareness.

Here's a fine example of a paradox with regards to every individual level of shielded self-awareness: you are your own unique expression of self-awareness (ego), who is the essence of your own present moment, yet, by being channelled through your physical soul (and brain), your good times and bad times approximate mere ripples in the flow of a cosmic presence. That's because in comparison to the cosmic mind, you're a shallower "droplet" of self-awareness. Once again, a deeper view on any type of dream world brings clarification. Understanding why time is self-awareness during a dream world makes clear why a deeper self is every dream soul, all at the same time.

A dream character channels a shallower level of shielded self-awareness owing to their soul's senses and sensations. In any type of a dream world, the dreamer is everyone ("every One"). The reason that a person can usually remember a dream world from only one point of view is because their deepest level of shielded self-awareness has the strongest connection with subconscious memory. That's why lucid awareness feels like being wide awake – while still being in the dream world.

Recently, after a particularly pleasant lucid dream, I wrote: "What gentle stream is reminding itself of being over-with the waterfall and pouring?" An answer arrived right away: such a gentle stream is a healthy stream of life. During a healthy dream's stream of life, shielded levels of the dreamer's self-awareness connect with healthy attitudes that make the dream world feel mighty good. While resonating within a stream of self-awareness that's harmonious with lucid love, you're capable of directing your dream world's subconscious energy in a healthy way. In the real world, the flow of self-awareness is more like a river of life, and this deeper river of life pours from an even greater and deeper presence of mind due to the immense connection!

We're each akin to one droplet in a great flowing river of self-awareness, and the same way a droplet of water can't be the river even though the river is every droplet, a person can't be their deepest self even though their deepest self is every person. What I mean is that although GOD is you, you're not GOD!

The waterfall symbolizes a tumultuous trauma blasting an ego into a disconnected droplet during dreams and in real life. At the bottom of the waterfall, you may endure a detached and egotistical viewpoint if you've impressed a belief in disconnection upon your subconscious mind, and you can really suffer.

A gentler flow of ego conscious appears to be powerfully peaceful because harmonious relationships with one another help to connect you with healthier states of subconscious energy. To all sorts of varying degrees, streams of life and rivers of life – and the spirit of life – are channelled by the calm pools and by the wild chaotic clamour of conscious and subconscious energy!

Although you always have a choice in which direction to take, every so often – similar to waterfalls – you're going to be flung downstream by your own subconscious mind. Of deeper significance, the "over-with the waterfall and pouring" part of that question: "What gentle stream is reminding itself of being over-with the waterfall and pouring?" symbolizes a pouring of lucid love. After you're over with the wild and chaotic clamour of your fall from the dizzying heights of an egotistical outlook, a gentle pouring of lucid love can channel healthy conscious energy through your subconscious mind.

When emotion flows from a heart filled with lucid love, conscious and subconscious energy come into balance. Parallel to healthy lucid dreaming, a balanced mind can channel happiness to life here in the real world!

Without understanding the real point of happiness, you may overlook every clue that solves the mystery of where your ego really comes from. A clueless outlook also enables your subconscious mind to feel fear! Feeling fear sets the stage for a tragic plunge into subconscious self-destruction; surely you've been there, done that, gone over the edge and off the deep end at some point in your life.

Going over the edge and off the deep end is really about the way egotistical thinking denies a loving relationship with the subconscious mind. A selfishly proud feeling of superiority can separate you from a more down to earth point of view. That's because people who consciously believe that their ego is a superior level of self-awareness become discordant due to the subconscious fear, anger, and hurt that goes along with such belief. While channelling a "waterfall" of disconnection into existence, people who believe in superior and inferior levels of self-awareness won't hesitate to bash, bully, or grab at anyone or anything when they hit bottom because they're drowning in drama!

Many people are unaware of a deeper point to life than just surviving shocking – and often traumatizing – drama. Selfishness and greed can lead the way for brutally dense thoughts to return even more nightmarish views. Egotistical thinking can justify harsh words and dirty deeds with new, narrow, and nasty attitudes.

Incredibly, sinister attitudes help save the cosmic mind from stagnating in tedious boredom! A waterfall of chaotic clamour turns out to be a backward fall helping to keep streams, rivers, and spirits of life moving onward. Then again, an ego who's loving the present moment directs their soul down a gentler stream of life that's "over-with the waterfall", and flowing merrily.

Lucid love reconnects conscious and subconscious energy with a happy outlook – a viewpoint that can free your soul from fear. Once again, the purpose of every individual level of self-awareness is to resist eternal boredom (and death). Nonetheless, lucid love reconnects a dotty ego!

## A Truer Meaning Of Happiness

Lucid dreaming demonstrates that self-awareness in a dream world and self-awareness in the real world have common connections. Unfortunately, talking about these connections doesn't seem so common! What's more, most folks ignore, forget, and even deny the significance of their dream worlds – haven't even thought about a deeper self, let alone respected one.

Noticing the parallels with dream worlds and the real world can ease long-term suffering coming from conscious belief in superiority and inferiority. For starters, you can step into a more comfortable presence of mind by trusting that every dimension of reality is an imaginary illusion taking place within a Great One Dreamer's subconscious mind.

Whenever you have a dream, a cosmic self experiences a dream within a dream. You're the deeper self for your dream souls because subconscious energy channels shallower levels of self-awareness, and in the same instant, your dream souls channel a greater cosmic self. In other words, the same Great One Dreamer is always One and all! This happens to be how and why, at a deeper rhythm of life, whether or not you realize it, we're all connected psychically in the here and now during dreams as well as in the real world. That's why stepping into a more connected presence of mind makes it possible for a person to become clairvoyant!

Stepping into a lucidly loving presence of mind also helps deeper clairvoyance – seeing what's not normally seen – to piece together a greater view on a truer meaning of happiness. A lucidly loving view enables you to toss old and unhealthy truth behind belief in unhappiness. Transforming an unhappy outlook into a healthier one helps you refine your ego's belief in self-definition.

Piecing together a basic view on a truer meaning of happiness can take place when you find your true self! Then again, truths are created from both healthy and unhealthy perception. A clearer look at the truest meaning of life helps you appreciate not only why perception creates belief in truth, "truth" also has an effect on perception!

You surely have some sort of truthful perception about who you believe you are, then again, there always comes that age old question: "What's the true meaning of life?" I hear lots of folks in our down to earth, real-world reality shouting out one answer with conviction: "The true meaning of life is money!"

Deep down in a human soul, a person's conscious belief in the power of money can make financial health feel like the most important truth of all! That's why you may believe that more money means more power to feel good. Going deeper in this direction of thought can make a person say that they feel like a million dollars if they're feeling good. Although this way of thinking doesn't produce a healthy viewpoint on such a serious topic as the true meaning of life, the perception does seem to be a common one. How you earn and spend your money can also have an effect on belief in self-definition. For a lot of folks, the honest truth is that with little or no money, you're inferior!

Throughout my younger days, I used a lot of my conscious and subconscious energy to try and earn a big income – which included paying my taxes! I believed that if enough people like me prospered financially, healthier communities could grow. Also, I thought that the type of job I held, the amount of cash I earned, and my materialistic possessions actually defined who I was. Unfortunately for me, I had a great deal of demanding work which wasn't much fun. Plus, topics of conversation on the job and at home were often about money, about who made the most by hurting the hardest. Along with my unhealthy duties at the pulp and paper mill power plants that I worked at in British Columbia, I felt plenty of anxiety, stress, and fear over what would happen if my "big" income stopped coming in. There were some good times too, although they seemed few and far between – until a deeper FTBT viewpoint began to redirect my outlook toward a healthier belief in a truer meaning of happiness.

Thanks to healthier lucid dream life, I eventually realized why a belief in the survival of the richest can really grind you down. That's because there's the suggestion that "Time is money!"

If you impress your subconscious soul with the notion that time is money, you're ruled by money and greed. It's healthier to believe that time is self-awareness because then a more wholesome spirit of life rules your subconscious. Since a greater spirit of life is the present moment, feeling a love for the present moment is loving all of life, and that's why giving love for life is a truer meaning of happiness.

If a truth behind belief in self-definition is based on an idea that you need lots of money in order to feel significant and useful, you're violating guidance from Lucid Law. The violation is due to a fear of not receiving, rather than loving life's game of giving and receiving. The Lucid Law of Belief serves to make clear how and why, if you expect things to happen a certain way due to your conscious belief, you're capable of bringing your expectation to life. If you expect to labour long and hard in order to make money, then your expectation is inharmonious with lucid love because your subconscious energy is bringing so much suffering into existence.

A belief in having to suffer in order to survive can actually separate you from what you truly want. Loving the present moment helps you escape from belief in having to hurt before you can ever feel good. If you view money as a way to escape from suffering, rather than as a reason to suffer, you can benefit from the ideas and understandings behind the Lucid Law of Belief. In other words, you won't get the right kind of deeper subconscious power to feel healthy happiness for the long-term if you won't love your own presence of mind.

That a belief in the amount of cash I'm worth in the real world is a measure for how happy I should feel seems silly from a lucidly loving point of view. A guiding principle behind the Lucid Law of Love – during any dimension of reality – is all about conscious belief in feeling good. Once again, if you believe that your money and the value of your assets are a measure for how happy you should feel, you can step away from a truer meaning of happiness.

If you can focus on how you really want to feel, you can clue into a bigger picture. This bigger picture includes understanding the ideas behind Lucid Law, which apply to everybody. If you expect to be wealthy, then you'll attract whatever makes you feel rich. But, if your words express a belief in poverty, then through the power of your subconscious mind, you can produce a truly poverty-stricken mood no matter how well-off you are.

A deeper question is: "What does a person really need in order to feel healthy happiness?" A tougher question! Once again, if you think about how you want to feel, then you might go along with the idea that you need to love the present moment in order to feel healthy happiness. More to the point, the high and mighty walls of your own financial inferiority – or financial superiority – can serve to isolate you from feeling a mood that's harmonious with lucid love.

More often than not, by comparing yourself against people higher up on the social ladder, you're capable of sliding into the types of attitudes that return moods of jealousy, and you may feel envious of those who appear wealthier. In such a state of affairs, your belief in being financially inferior can slip you away from feeling good; however, along with the lucidly loving mindset that arrives from comprehending all seven lucid laws, you're capable of transforming an unhappy mood. Through a deeper thinking, real-world outlook, you can get some real subconscious power to feel long-lasting happiness by feeding your cosmic mind some lucid love!

Going along with the Lucid Law of Love's guidance for feeling healthy happiness gets you some wisdom to realize why a higher cash flow doesn't make any one person superior to another. Money is important, but there's a healthier way to get really rich: love the present moment! Lucid dreaming and lucid awareness serve to show how and why your truer self during any dream world is far greater than just a "flesh and blood" dream body, an inner voice, or a separate attitude. In every type of a dream world, your true self is everyone's self-awareness. Additionally, no amount of cash is required to step your dream world into a happy mood. And, it's the same deal in the real world because whatever you consciously believe, you make feel real.

A campaign to make lucid love the healthy truth behind the real meaning of happiness can be helpful to one and all thanks to the wholesome world view. That's because a lucidly loving point of view respects and cares about everyone. This way, instead of fearing that you're going to receive more of whatever makes you feel poor, a conscious belief in your own deeper self being everybody's deeper self enables you to realize that healthy happiness can't be bought – it's given.

## CHAPTER EIGHT

# FREEDOM FROM FEAR OF FEAR

Not long after those recurring medieval dreams (described in chapter two) took place, another pivotal lucid dream helped me realize the difference between healthy and unhealthy truth. This healthy lucid dream was key for my freedom from unhealthy belief in fear of fear! The dream began with me standing in a place that was super quiet; I focused on the silence. Along with a perfectly peaceful atmosphere, a quick look around showed aisles filled with shelves upon shelves that supported fantastic looking models of eighteenth century era warships.

My first glance around the place brought me some splendid perception. Since still being a bit of a history buff, my admiration for this shop was far beyond what would be usual. Built with such intricate detail, these models appeared miraculous to me! Plus, I noticed price tags on the ships and there were lots of zeros after the numbers. Their actual cost wasn't what enlivened me, delightful surprise made me feel really good!

The store appeared to be long standing. A rich Turkey carpet covered the floor, felt plush beneath my stocking feet. Low walls were made of dark wood panelling; a white-painted plaster ceiling was only a hands width above my head. The atmosphere of the place was solemn and preserved, like a museum.

At the beginning of the <u>Ship Shop</u> lucid dream, I wasn't in a lucid level of self-awareness. Along with my consciously believing that I was in a real shop, I merely wandered around the place, admiring beautiful looking replicas of square-rigged British, French, American, and Spanish warships; there appeared to be several dozen throughout the store, and some looked to be over two meters in length. While I was standing in an aisle filled with shelves full of these amazing works of art on either side of me, I saw some people at the far end of my walkway – three very old looking women sat at a small round table. Drizzle blurred my view through the window behind them, but outside there appeared to be a cobblestone street that was deserted.

I looked more closely at the little old ladies who were setting down dainty tea cups. Three elderly souls were placing their cups on the small round table. Repositioning of crockery brought forth waves of tinkling that cut up the deep silence. In addition, two of the old gals seemed to be smiling at me. That's why I walked right up to their table, while smiling back.

Of course, I couldn't record the exact conversation in my dream diary; however, my impression of our extensive chat was an eye-opener! The nearest woman kept smiling while slowly standing from her chair. With her head down and shoulders forward, she turned sideways, peeked up at me and said, "William, so nice to meet you, I'm Anna."

Anna appeared to be a conventional "little old lady" except that her wispy hair, which was shoulder length, was bright white – like pure snow in sunshine. She put a hand out, palm down, and I automatically bowed before her. Next, I knelt on one knee, took her extended hand into both of mine and gently kissed her bony knuckles.

Anna giggled, pointed with her other hand at an even older looking woman and said, "This is Annabelle."

Annabelle made her way, unhurriedly, into a crooked standing posture. I changed position, kissed one of Annabelle's hands, and she nodded her head a little. I noticed that beneath Annabelle's wide-brimmed hat, her face was expressionless. Her eyes looked large, and were set well apart, but they stared straight ahead. I wondered if she might be blind.

Once again, Anna pointed and said, "This is Kathleen." The third aged woman displayed a lively looking smile, but remained seated. Kathleen was in a wheelchair. She leaned forward, presented her hand to be kissed. After the formality, Kathleen turned her palm up to reveal a dazzling looking ruby ring! The ruby was the size of a walnut, the ring a thick band of gold. Kathleen slipped the heavy ring onto my wedding finger and as she spoke, her voice carried a tone of kindness: "You've earned this ruby for all these beautiful ships here in our shop – good work William."

I whispered, "Thanks."

At this point, I suddenly realized that I was in a dream world! I felt as though a mind restricting shield was abruptly lifted away, enabling me to understand that my subconscious mind had created all the beautiful model ships in this wonderful shop. I was the One accountable for everything because my presence of mind was the entire dream world.

After fully aligning, connecting, and merging with my real-world ego conscious, there came a rush of excitement due to my realization of being in a dream world. A quick pinch on my forearm – and the accompanying feeling of dull numbness – had me trusting that I was in a different dimension of reality!

Kathleen grinned at me and said, "Sit down with us William – we've got some important things to talk about." She leaned back in her wheelchair, and I wondered if the low creak came from the wheelchair, or from her. Kathleen was thin and frail looking, yet, her facial expressions were still lively. What's more, she wore a polished and eye-catching pearl necklace which hung loosely around her navy blue, turtleneck sweater!

I sat down on a straight back wooden chair beside their small round table, bowed my head, and focused on the richly coloured Turkey carpet in order to remain calm. After what felt like a moment in eternity, I tuned into the sound of Anna and Annabelle working their way back into their seats. Also admiring the stunning ring on my finger, I said to myself, "This ring is so stunning! If only I could bring it back home. Not very likely since home is in another dimension of reality where only my self-awareness may return. Calm… remain calm. Breathe deep and slow. Give love to the present moment. Ah well, after some tea, I'm definitely going to check out all the rest of the ships in this amazing shop. They look so real!"

Next, I detected Kathleen's lively tone of voice – heard her say rather loudly, "William! Ahoy William, are you here to free yourself from unhealthy truths?" Her aristocratic English accent was sharp.

"Huh?", I murmured. My mind left the luxury of the ring, and I remember feeling surprised at the depth of Kathleen's query. A dream character who spoke about unhealthy truth was extraordinary! I returned my focus of attention onto the Turkey carpet between my feet, but also zoomed in on the sound of her voice.

Kathleen continued, "Let me explain… a person's truths come from the way their existence is perceived. That's why, if someone gives a healthy smile, they're usually feeling a pleasing perception. It's all a loop. Healthy truth is linked with fearless and loving belief while unhealthy truth is linked with fearful and resentful belief, but either way, a cycle is set in motion."

Kathleen paused, and with my head still bowed down I asked, "A cycle? What kind of a cycle do you mean?"

After finally breaking my focus off the carpet beneath my feet, I brought my head up to gaze respectfully at the sweetest smile on Kathleen's elderly face. Then she said, "Truths cycle up and down, back and forth, round and round with attitudes, and that's why attitudes drive cyclic loops. These loops are what we want to talk about. That's because they're Karmic. Karmic loops are central to the idea of destiny. You can cope with these loops a lot more easily when you understand what's really going on: it's those events you pay attention to, and just as importantly, those you choose to ignore that bring about coping strategies."

I said, "OK, for sure it's what you pay true and profound attention to that gets noticed – unless what you're not noticing comes back and bites you!"

Kathleen said, "Yes, you can get blindsided by your own Karma – sorry dear Annabelle – she's blind you know William."

"Oh never you mind," piped in Annabelle, her tone of voice smooth as silk, "It's my honest intention to believe in healthy truth and happy emotion since truths behind beliefs are what fill the Karma loops. That's why I'm happy, even though I'm blind."

I went along with her idea by saying, "Uh huh, yeah… healthy truth is important, but what has all this got to do with model ships in a ship shop?" My questioning voice was calm.

From the shadow beneath the brim of Annabelle's sunhat, her wide eyes stared straight ahead as she said, "These ships define a truth behind your belief in fear."

The blank look on Annabelle's puffed and wrinkled face was at odds with her active mind. After a sip of tea, she continued: "I know we may all look and sound a little loopy... oh hmm ha, ha! But, when you can focus on what you believe feels fearful, you can begin to recognize where your fear comes from; then, you may figure out the underlying truth behind it all. That's why you need to pay attention to your feelings – realize what feels real, and just as importantly, pay attention to your idea of truth!

I sipped on my cup of hot tea, and oh my, it tasted so good! A dainty tea cup had appeared in front of me, and the tea was going down nicely.

All the while, Anna's slightly higher pitched voice was saying: "Feeling good about an unhealthy truth can happen when you intend to get some revenge. If you believe that a person has committed an injustice, you may feel good about making the person suffer." Her wispy, snow-white hair framed her sunken eyes, jutting chin, and lightly moving lips. She also said, "Although a vengeful attitude may make you feel a burst of unhealthy happiness, the unhealthy truth is that such belief channels Karmic loops that don't feel good in the long run."

I caught the drift of where this conversation was headed – the real warships that the models replicated were intended to contend with hostile environments. Perhaps there was another contentiousness, another argument for noble bursts of brute force feeling good, but in an unhealthy way? I suddenly remembered the "noble" knights from my medieval dreams. Those dreams were always crossing my mind. I cut short the calm silence settling in at our table and blurted, "Oh for sure a truth may be unhealthy even though it can feel good, just like the way a selfishly proud knight first felt during a medieval dream I had!"

Anna and Kathleen glanced at each other with raised eyebrows.

"Medieval dream?" asked Annabelle. Her faraway eyes gazed straight ahead. "You were in medieval times?"

"Well, kind of... you see, I had some recurring dreams that revolved around a medieval village – I mean this old-fashioned village felt like it had been there forever!" I suddenly realized that my comments about agedness might offend these aged dream characters. Same as in the real world, in dream worlds a sharp comment can be perceived as hurtful. I glanced at each face and felt relieved – there were no hard stares, nor stiff frowns.

Then Kathleen, the one who gave me the astonishing ruby ring asked: "What were you doing in a medieval village, dearest William?" Kathleen's wheelchair was gone. She was sitting upon a throne! Studded with sparkling emeralds, her new high-back chair looked as though it were made of solid gold. Although Kathleen's frail looking head still protruded from her navy blue turtleneck sweater (and the polished pearl necklace was still there), she was now enveloped in scarlet coloured cushioning.

I said, "At first I was a serf, and I felt terrified! My focus was on the action taking place around me. Internally, I was experiencing a freeze response."

"A what?" asked Anna. "What in the world is a cheese response?"

While glancing up at the plaster ceiling, Kathleen sighed.

I turned away from Kathleen to look at Anna, and spoke loudly: "Not cheese. A freeze response means that your muscles become rigid. When a person, or any conscious animal is in mortal danger, automatic responses kick in. You know, it's the old fight or flight thing."

"Or freeze," added Annabelle in a kindly manner. "Comes from mortal fear. Fight, flight, or freeze. Everyone always forgets about the freeze bit."

Anna grinned, and while nodding her head up and down, she uttered, "Oh yes it's alright William, I get it now. It's these old ears you know, they don't hear as well as they used to!"

This time Annabelle sighed; Kathleen merely rolled her eyes.

I continued: "Anyway, even though everything was just a dream, I was so scared that I couldn't move, could hardly breathe. Of course I didn't know that I was in a dream world. I thought everything was real. I honestly believed that I was going to die because at first, fighting great huge knights wasn't an option. Those medieval dreams were also about the deeper power of true fear!"

Annabelle said, "Oh right you are there, William. But, do you see what we're really talking about?" Now blind Annabelle was asking me if I could see. After a slight pause she continued: "A fearful attitude returns Karmic loops with more disturbing perception seeming true as true can be."

"Oh yeah!" I blurted. Then I said, "While they were happening, I believed that those medieval nightmares were real!"

"Yes, yes." whispered Annabelle. "Not only that, you can continue to feel offended, and give offence, in fearful ways. Resentful Karmic loops return from real fear. Fear fills unhealthy Karmic loops."

I looked around the table and felt much respect for such words of wisdom. "Yes," I said, "And that's why if there's no way to fight back, and no escaping, then you'll automatically slip into a freeze response."

I was beginning to realize that some sort of deeper point was coming; I kept talking in order to ready myself. I spoke quickly, with a full recall of my real-world training in hypnotherapy: "This fearful energy arriving from a belief in mortal death, it can instantly induce a type of trance state. Similar to the way a nerve becomes frozen by a dentist's unthinking needle, a person's intuitive, yet, unthinking subconscious mind can freeze their soul's entire nervous system to numb potential pain. In other words, while you impress your subconscious mind with a conscious belief in imminent death, you won't feel any physical pain – until afterwards, if your soul survives!"

I finished up by adding: "The freeze response actually does a double duty because a predator may think you're dead, and leave you alone for a while."

"A predator!" exclaimed Annabelle, "Like a shark?"

"Or a thug," whispered Kathleen.

"A beast!" announced Anna.

We all nodded in agreement. After a sobering measure of the intimate moment I said, "If there's a chance to escape or fight back, you can awaken from your trance state and take action. All sorts of creatures shake, shudder, and tremble as though thawing out after experiencing a life-threatening event. If the injury wasn't fatal, a surviving wild animal can carry on without the burden of resentment whereas with a person, attitudes seem way more complicated."

Anna nodded her head up and down while saying, "That's so true! Major problems can follow – if you're unable or unwilling to let go of a resentful attitude. An angry Karma loop turns a narrower groove that's hard to break out of.

Then Annabelle said, "Am I hearing you say that you can get shocked and traumatized from belief in a fear of fear?"

I answered confidently, "A traumatized human soul comes from their ego's ongoing perception of fear."

From her throne, Kathleen said, "That's the key – ongoing fear comes from conscious belief; a soul can continue to get shocked by conscious energy. A healthy way to shake off such shock is to weep. Shuddering and trembling from weeping – without fear – can transform shocked and hurtful subconscious energy. Sobbing changes a Karmic loop!"

"Ah yes," I said, "I think I see what you're getting at. A release from fear can come about when you impress your subconscious mind with healthy truth that your deeper self has been forgiven. Babies and young children do it all the time – you see and hear their crying and bawling as though the world were coming to an end; then, two minutes later, they can be truly loving the moment again!"

From her golden throne, Kathleen said, "For the young and the old, fear can provide a powerful adrenaline rush to fight, flee, or freeze into place in order to survive a situation perceived as life threatening. The situation isn't what creates an adrenaline rush – a perception of the situation creates the rush. For one thing, you may not even notice anything until it's too late. It's conscious belief in your situation being truly fearful that can instantly generate a bodily feeling of fear."

Kathleen looked me in the eye with an intenseness matched by the passion in her voice. She made her point clear by saying, "So, just as you said, surviving a fearful perception of an event doesn't always bring closure to the impact of your own shock. Without transforming your original subconscious memory of having been shocked, you're unable to escape from unhealthy emotion, and unhealthy Karmic loops keep you spinning in circles of suffering!"

Annabelle picked up the pace, "Belief in fear can drive unhealthy moods. With an unhealthy mood in place, your world follows patterns where you get more shocked energy streaming from the original traumatic response. In due course, you may feel anxiously stressed all the time!"

Annabelle took a moment to catch her breath, and I got the chance to ask, "Wait a sec, are you talking about dream worlds, or real-life stuff?"

"Does it matter?" asked Annabelle. "We're talking about emotion. You may believe that you're caught up in a nightmare, that the harder you try to escape, the worse things get. Did this happen in your medieval dreams?

Did your own voice freeze because conscious belief had you feeling so fearful?"

"Yes," I answered somewhat sheepishly, "And when I was the knight in shining armour, I was actually feeling pretty good with my belief in superiority, although now that you mention it, I recognize how I was feeling happy in an unhealthy way, just like a beast."

"Poor dear William," said Anna. "Conscious belief in superiority can have you condemning those creatures that you perceive to be inferior. Then again, belief in inferiority can bring you a mind numbing fear of those whom you believe are superior!"

Annabelle quipped, "This makes our final point – fear stems from conscious belief that may not be healthy. Many people feel terrified by mice, spiders, garden snakes, open spaces, confined spaces, heights, or crowds to mention but a few. You can experience an extreme anxiety complex because of the deeper truth behind a perception."

"This is so important," added Kathleen, "When a belief gets defined by fearful, angry, and hurtful perception, unhealthy truth can transform a person's level of self-awareness. This way, the unhealthy truth that you believe in is what you get, no matter how imaginary."

Annabelle said, "Just watch the news on television for a few minutes! Great masses of people have based many of their conscious beliefs on the fearful points of view coming from ugly news on their televisions. Instead of looking inward and adjusting an unhealthy truth, how many times do you choose to ignore, deny, and forget about alternative perception that conflicts with fearful belief?"

Kathleen finished up by saying, "What we're trying to tell you is that you can become trapped in an unhealthy viewpoint! When truth is unhealthy, you lose control over your own subconscious energy. Until the day you die, your world view conforms to the real truth behind your belief."

"Wow," was all I could say. There was more to the truth behind a belief than I'd realized!

We stayed quiet for a while, and during the resonating sound of silence, I pondered upon the real truth behind my belief in fear. I finally stood from the table and said, "I'll think about all your words of wisdom while I look around, if that's OK?"

"By all means," replied Anna, "Take your time, enjoy."
Kathleen nodded with a smile and said, "Bye for now Wiilliam."
Annabelle called out, "Toodles."

I left their cozy table, wandered around to the next aisle where right away, I paused to scrutinize a gorgeous looking triple-decker – a first-rate British battleship! As I stared into her rigging, the ship came alive; on a scale proportional with the ship's size, there were hundreds of tiny sailors, and they were moving! This lucid dream still had a long way to go. In the end, the ship would let loose with a full broadside – a thundering cannonade coming from every proud sailor's conscious belief in the truth of superior firepower!

## Firewalker

Thanks to the <u>Ship Shop</u> lucid dream, I stepped toward a healthier presence of mind. Daring to face a firewalker event freed me from a fearful view on superior firepower! There may be sudden occasions when focusing attention on a fearful view of reality can help a person survive while in a nasty Karmic loop. The three basic critical emotions involved with bad Karma – fear, anger, and hurt – may be appropriate, yet, contentious emotions capable of warning you about your subconscious mind being impressed by belief in unhealthy truth.

Fifteen folks attended the firewalker event: it took place at a friend's place – a healthy house with several acres of property – out in the Sannich Peninsula countryside, just outside the city of Victoria, on Vancouver Island. My wife and I were the first to arrive there since I'd promised to build the fire. My wife came along only to watch. She kept talking about how there was no way she would ever walk through a fire! Plus, she'd promised her mother to oppose another of my untamed adventures; her honest intention was to talk me out of the whole thing.

While driving our car into the countryside, I went on and on about how my intention was only to get the fire going. I wanted to make sure there would be no tricks because I also believed a safe walk through a real fire would be impossible.

We arrived in the early afternoon. After a warm welcome, I got my chainsaw out of the car, built a huge fire! There were lots of old logs, branches – even a pile of firewood on the property. Not only did a nice bit of the backyard get cleaned up, no one could get near it for several hours! The sky darkened long before the fire burned low enough for anyone to approach. A calm, cool evening was at odds with the inflamed back yard.

Eventually, I raked red hot embers into a path which was about two meters wide and six meters long; the crimson coloured cinders were so hot that the handle on my rake kept bursting into flames! I said to myself: "No one could possibly walk this walk." Then I began to wonder if perhaps my wife and her mother were correct – maybe this was a foolish exploit after all; meanwhile, we still had Shawn, a most amazing and clever group leader.

Shawn arrived at the back yard soon after the fire's searing residue was raked into place. Shawn was short and chubby, always appeared to be a jolly fellow. This evening, he wore a fancy light blue, three-piece suit. In addition, an indigenous Canadian Indian accompanied him. His helper was tall and slim, wore traditional swayed leather pants and jacket, a feather head-dress – carried a large drum. Shawn said hello to everyone while the indigenous fellow banged on his ancient looking drum.

Shawn requested that everyone remove their shoes and socks before gathering for the fire walk. Barefoot, eleven out of the original fifteen – including me and my wife – crowded close. Shawn and his helper stood between us and the fire, which blazed sporadically into the night sky. My wife told me that she was alongside to make sure I wouldn't get hurt. She also said that she felt really scared!

Shawn asked us all to hold hands, close our eyes, and repeat his words. My wife held one of my hands while the other was clasped by another woman there to participate; both my hands were clenched in ironclad grips!

Shawn's chanting went on and on about channelling a group frame of mind that could transcend physical limitation here in the real world. Shawn's tone of voice, his rhythmic words, along with his helper's steady drumming and humming were dehypnotizing – I felt as though my fear of the fire walk was melting into the embers. A closer connection with a greater group presence made me recognize that yes, being here was very much like being in a dreamlike moment. Plus, the tight hand gripping had relaxed.

Finally, Shawn stepped toward the beginning (or end) of the glowing pathway; then, he stomped across the red hot coals! He walked all the way from one end to the other and came out smiling. After that, he turned his back to us and showed the bottom of each bare foot – not a mark!

I felt thrilled! Immediately, we all let go of each other's hands. I headed toward the same end of the fire where Shawn had entered, but my wife got there first! She was the second person to stomp over the burning coals. I made my incredible journey after she crossed safely. I took six large strides forward, and was through. I checked my feet – no pain, no blisters, not even a mark. Almost everyone made the crossing at least once – I made two, and my wife went an incredible three times!

Although originally talking the talk, and being there to participate, those few folks who refused to walk the walk seemed not to be believing their own eyes. Too frightened to test new insight, the people with "contentiously" resistive attitudes seemed to be frozen in their lonely abandonment. Instead of connecting with the harmonious joy that we firewalkers felt after having dehypnotized our subconscious energy from fear, their worried looking facial expressions revealed levels of consciousness that weren't loving the present moment. These folks stayed trapped in their conscious belief about the honest truth of what should've taken place – a bunch of fools getting their feet burnt off!

The firewalker event made me realize a healthier truth. That's because a healthy respect for firepower needn't include feeling terrified. By consciously believing that your real world is similar to another dimension of dreaming, you can view a truly threatening person, ferocious animal, fantastic firewalker event, or even a cannonade with respect instead of fear.

During the firewalker event, we firewalkers trusted in a healthy group connection. Since Shawn didn't get burnt, neither would we. The new belief in firewalking still included the old perception of a blazing danger, but only up to a certain point. There wasn't so much judgement about what should take place – there was more flow with what was taking place.

Afterwards, the non-participants expressed their belief that the fire was somehow rigged! But, I knew that it was all real. How can a person step out of fear? A simple answer is: intend to love the present moment!

Sooner than later, healthy truth behind loving (and respecting) the present moment channels harmonious joy, lucid love, and delightful surprise! While consciously believing that every living soul is here to toss a cosmic mind's state of eternal boredom, there really is a "truer" meaning to life. Resisting boredom in a lucidly loving way helps you transcend fear! This way, your smile may glow with healthy happiness because your bad Karma stops recurring. Once again, there happens to be a possibility for you to imagine real life as being a beautiful new dream, rather than an ugly old nightmare.

Windows of self-awareness in the real world are similar to windows of self-awareness taking place during dream worlds because the same deeper self looks through all windows at the same time. Clearly, along with conscious belief to care about your deeper self in dream worlds, you can dare to notice and care about a cosmic self – here and now – in the real world too!

# CHAPTER NINE

# CONSCIOUS AND SUBCONSCIOUS BALANCE

Proven pearls of wisdom pouring from lucid dreaming point out why the "true" meaning of life – to toss eternal boredom for a cosmic mind – can feel really good! Yet, trying to transform an unhappy subconscious mood may be a long and complicated journey; however, a lucidly loving pathway to freedom is a fast paced, quick, and easy way to go.

Bringing conscious and subconscious energy into balance happens to be a lot more straightforward if you can tune into six special points of view that flow with guidance from the Lucid Law of Tossing your Burden. This way, an egotistical attitude may be tossed. Tossing an egotistical attitude can transform an unhappy subconscious mood because a deathlike fading of selfishness and greed brings a state of emotional and mental stability in which a person is calm and able to make rational decisions.

Guidance from the Lucid Law of Tossing Your Burden enables six special points of view to mesh with lucid love, bringing conscious and subconscious energy into balance – easily. This different way of thinking avoids subconscious fear over a change in conscious belief because such an unconventional direction of thought balances conscious respect with subconscious compassion for ignorant attitudes.

The six special points of view are like six powerful lifeboats, each capable of rescuing you from drowning in unhappiness. That's because a buoyant level of self-awareness can channel a deeper thinking outlook! This new school of thought uses useful reasoning to make healthy and long-lasting happiness resonate within your soul. And speaking of useful, here comes number one of the six!

## Useful

The first of the six special points of view is all about the idea that when you feel useful, you can feel good. A good mood returns a useful attitude because such a mood adds value and benefit for your soul and for the cosmic soul – the fabric for a physical universe. You may fulfil your deepest purpose – to toss the cosmic mind's boredom – in a harmoniously happy way, a direction that you want to keep going in.

Feeling useful is of vital importance for flowing with lucid love and greater subconscious power because while feeling a conscious connection with a deeper purpose, any bleak clouds of uselessness may be blown away, easily. So, what describes the most useful thing that every person does? Continuing to "feel" reality from an individualistic point of view in order to consciously believe that such a place is real presents a rational answer.

The purpose of real life reality is to realize different levels of self-awareness – in order to toss ultimate boredom; besides, impressing harmoniously joyful, lucidly loving, as well as delightfully surprising energy upon your soul is most useful because this way, you can feel good. While feeling healthy happiness, your subconscious soul breathes life into an existence that you can love.

In due course, an ego must also experience fear, anger, and hurt in order to appreciate the difference between good and bad moods. But, if you get stuck in a shadowy life of shady intentions, your own subconscious soul can continue to intensify a nightmarish mood since you're capable of creating Karmic loops of crap!

Thinking from a level of lucid awareness during a lucid dream world makes me believe that every dream soul helps deepen a miraculous and wondrous dimension of usefulness – dreaming! In the real world, a deeper sensation of usefulness can be difficult to discover because there's only a tiny minority of us – soon to increase – who understand how and why every seemingly individual soul is the same dreamer.

Thankfully, you may consciously believe that self-awareness in the real world is similar to self-awareness in your dream worlds, and that's because all of existence is a dimension of conscious and subconscious energy. Understanding why a cosmic mind lives every level of self-awareness – all at the same time – in dream worlds and here in the real world, automatically steps you into the majority when it comes down to realizing a truer meaning of life!

Although the true meaning of life – to toss a state of eternal boredom – is the same for all life forms, most people seem to give the impression of feeling unsympathetic when feeding on live (like a livewire) energy. Yet, an intention to love sharing the present moment you're helping create can bring you a valid reason for drawing the line on your cosmic self having to suffer with so much pain and misery in order to toss boredom. Transforming any living soul into food for thought challenges the idea of giving lucid love because the present moment includes the self-awareness of all people as well as all of nature.

A clear intention to support worldwide logging, mining, hunting, fishing, and farming industries in order to support a worldwide human population explosion is an example of a major challenge for giving lucid love. These global activities may help build the infrastructure necessary for increasing the quality of your home, town, and city life, but a lot of folks don't seem to care about the extent of change – and suffering – taking place for levels of subconscious energy due to such commotion. You probably don't want to be a person who's unwilling to walk upon the grass because of a concern for harming the environment; nevertheless, a healthy truth behind loving the present moment is to care about deep stepping footprints.

While human beings annihilate the natural world in order to channel a more materialistic and artificial environment, you can still believe in usefulness by remembering how the real world may be viewed as another dimension of dreaming. During a dream world, your deeper self can't really be killed; albeit, burning or harvesting old growth trees while tossing forest and jungle life can transmit traumatic consequences for conscious and subconscious energy in any dimension of reality! In spite of this, you may continue to believe in your own soul's usefulness while benefiting from such a transformation of the environment, owing to a clear intention for survival rather than greed.

An increasing human population is in direct proportion to the rate of environmental realignment taking place. Environmental realignment is a transformation of the surrounding ("environ") and mentally aware ("mental") energy. A trade-off for more human life is less forest, jungle, sea, and lake life. So, are we going to reach a tipping point where the planet's human population eventually dies out owing to an unhealthy transformation of the natural world? Not necessarily!

Giving lucid love can help turn the tide on the natural world's unhealthy transformation. Individual levels of self-awareness channelled by trees, plants, birds, bugs, fish, animals, and all other nonhuman souls are being transformed at an alarming rate in order to feed, clothe, and shelter an increasing number of human souls; meanwhile, although people's egotistical outlooks are widespread, experiencing a boring dimension of real-life reality isn't on the horizon!

A deeper look into the Lucid Law of Tossing Your Burden makes clear that a healthy balance for a little conscious energy is a lot of subconscious energy! Instead of more wars, an ongoing global pandemic, or an all out Armageddon, a global intention to reduce the number of people on the planet – from a lucidly loving outlook – is a more caring path for healthy conscious and subconscious balance. You can be part of a global intention to invent (and discover) new technology that'll get humanity's physical souls to another planet! People can physically explore a greater subconscious universe and expand consciousness!

Populating a spiral galaxy – the Milky Way – would be a good way to sustain a spiralling human population. But, does anybody really want to live on the Moon, on Mars, or in a spaceship? If you're loving the moment, then yes! First, we could just toss the seeds. A spaceship could be filled with soil, seeds, and all the programming required to plant new life on another planet that has water!

Travelling into the solar system could create new stepping stones toward expanded levels of consciousness. At any rate, a soaring number of human souls are capable of channelling deeper consciousness from a greater subconscious soul – the cosmic universe – thanks to conscious belief that healthy usefulness is an important part of a lucidly loving viewpoint.

## Thankful

Thankfulness is another of the six special points of view that flow with guidance from the Lucid Law of Tossing Your Burden. When I realize I'm dreaming, I feel thankful for being in a different dimension of reality. Also, I feel grateful for the awareness that I can't really be injured or killed! Intending to keep on feeling grateful for having consciousness in a fantasy that feels real helps the lucid dream flow in a healthy direction. While my lucid dream world is flowing in a healthy direction, I feel healthy happiness.

Thankfulness for the idea that everyone's deeper self is the same spirit of life – a Great One Dreamer (GOD) who purposely dreams real-life reality into existence – can feel real. When such thankfulness is believable, it becomes subconscious. Subconscious thankfulness for having a human life returns moods filled with healthy happiness. Intending to keep on feeling grateful for being part of a cosmic moment directs the real world time continuum in a lucidly-loving direction.

Feeling thankful for whatever dimension of reality you're experiencing – here and now – is a healthy conscious connection with the cosmic mind. You can brighten your own window of self-awareness, thanks to a lucidly loving attitude. A lucidly loving attitude is filled with thankfulness from a conscious realization that ultimate boredom has been tossed in a healthy way!

The deeper you can focus on believing in thankfulness, the more you can find to feel thankful for. Lots of warm-hearted laughter and healthy smiles go a long way toward helping you feel thankful for tossing boredom in healthy ways. Feeling thankful for the greater one present moment that we're all experiencing is capable of stepping you into a breathtaking and brilliant dimension of consciousness this very instant, right now!

Thankfulness gets you grounded in a deeper love for life. That's because when you're grounded in lucid love, you can understand why unhealthy truth may override and even cancel out thankfulness. Healthy truth behind thankfulness brings balance to conscious and subconscious energy. Yet, an unbalanced mind can pull the curtain down on your own window of self-awareness because with a heavily guarded attitude in place, you can deny who you really are – everyone and everything!

Whether you believe that you're more important than those around you, or you view relatives, friends, team-mates, community, or even your entire country as separate and superior, you're able to get caught up in the selfish rush of egotism. Selfishly proud attitudes can bring you into a greedy presence of mind. Along with proud emotion from belief in your soul's ego being better than another soul's ego, feeling thankful for everyone being of equal significance isn't going to happen – that's why we have the old saying that pride always precedes a fall. Eventually, you'll splash down from your "waterfall" of departure, and the final crash can feel terrifying!

The unhealthy truth behind a belief in selfish pride builds wicked walls of separation and inharmonious shielding between an ego and the subconscious mind. For example: you might believe that a person can feel proud about something as innocent as thinking that their national flag is the best flag in the world. Pride feels similar to thankfulness at the start, but pride is a different emotion than gratitude. With pride framing your window of self-awareness, the view can get really twisted!

You may untwist and toss a selfishly proud viewpoint by simply using the word "thankful" instead of "proud" while expressing thoughts. Instead of proclaiming that you're proud to be from a country that you believe is better than any other, a healthier viewpoint is all about giving thanks that all nationality is precious. Words are magical because an entire dimension of reality can be loved or abused by what you say since the subconscious mind is always listening.

Expressing gratitude for the idea that a cosmic mind is every level of self-awareness, all at the same time, is another way to toss egotism and selfish pride. Feeling thankful for tossing your deeper self's boredom helps bring you into a lucidly loving outlook. Being part of a network of supporting friends in a joyful and loving environment may not always be possible, but if your window of self-awareness frames even one heartbeat of respect for a thankful point of view, your mood can soar with healthy happiness.

## **Respectful**

A healthy mood may be felt when you respect the idea that the true meaning of life is all about a cosmic self's (GOD's) escape from eternal boredom. Respecting your presence of mind – your present moment – brings about another of the special points of view that lead to feeling real respect for the good, the bad, and the ugly!

Feeling respect for a peek at ultimate subconscious power reveals another way to resonate with lucid love. That is, all souls are of value since every living soul helps toss ultimate power's greatest burden – eternal boredom. When you respect all levels of self-awareness, you're showing respect for your present moment.

Respect for an escape from eternal boredom helps float a lucidly loving outlook. An ego is capable of tossing selfish and greedy attitudes. The challenge of facing up to egotism – whether contending with your own egotistical attitudes, or those of another bully – were discussed throughout chapter seven, and deeper subconscious power from showing respect is also revealed there. Not only that, as far as deeper subconscious power is concerned, emotions aren't able to think. Gut instinct, moral belief, and a means for survival can conflict as you toss selfish greed; however, decisions followed by seemingly appropriate actions must occur. For instance: people need to eat and drink in order to stay alive!

If you search for food in local markets, a lucidly loving outlook can make you realize that food markets sell subconscious energy! Justification for transforming another living soul into food for thought comes from a respect for your own soul's state of health – you must consume live energy in order to keep your soul healthy and your own individual ego surviving. Yet, when you see those small aquariums where untamed conscious souls such as lobsters and crabs are kept for many days and nights – piled on top of one another – before being taken and boiled alive, you're witnessing some hauntingly evil disrespect for the present moment.

A lucidly loving outlook includes considerate and respectful views on the idea that shielded levels of the same self-awareness are channelled by all life forms – including people whose attitudes are afflicted with egotism! Lucid love floats to life when you feel healthy respect for the idea that all levels of self-awareness add up to give the present moment direction!

The next time you're eating, you may consider the idea that eating in moderation shows respect for the live energy you're consuming.

## Healthy

A rosy and comfy mood arrives with the fourth of the six special buoying points of view – your physical and financial health! A healthy attitude and healthy soul are harmonious with one another, and are fundamental for a happy mood. Lucid love also progresses with a happy mood since once again, you can make your real world feel like a healthy dream world when you toss boredom in a way that's harmonious with loving your presence of mind.

Healthier dimensions of reality arrive with wholesome outlooks on life; nevertheless, a lot of egotistically minded people have such fragmented outlooks that their thoughts and actions can seem suicidal! Clearly, an idea to commit suicide doesn't come from a wholesome outlook on life, unless, if suddenly infected with a fatal and contagious syndrome (and facing painful bodily death), you might want to "pinch out" ahead of "time". Sacrifice might also feel necessary while staying in a lethal environment in order to help shut down potentially perilous machinery such as a malfunctioning nuclear power plant, inevitably saving a community. In rare cases like these, a person may believe that suicide and self-sacrifice are healthy choices. The thing is, why else would anyone intentionally kill their soul? One huge reason comes from an egotistical plunge into drama.

If your financial life is in ruin because you've no money, you're capable of hitting rock bottom too hard. Unable to cope with so much self implosion, you may ask yourself: "What's the point of it all?" Egotistical thoughts can set severe whining tones to internal and external complaining. A person's mood may get so ugly that pinching out (committing suicide) might seem like the only path for ending overwhelming suffering. You may be plagued with injury and disease as your soul begins to open death's door – due to being impressed with conscious belief that all of existence is all about suffering. And sometimes, during a period of extreme self-loathing, committing suicide may be the final episode of a real-life nightmare because hating the present moment creates the most fragmented outlook of all time!

Real suffering arrives from a closed-minded belief that there's no deeper spiritual connection with the present moment – an unhealthy truth that can eventually make your outlook fearful. If you complain about your present moment being rotten, you're impressing an underlying belief in rot upon your own soul. Unawareness that your spirit of life is the present moment can bring about long-lasting bad moods, physical disease, and mental illness because you may be blindsided by bad Karma.

## The Angel Lucid Dream

The <u>Angel</u> lucid dream taught me how some common types of rot can creep into a soul. This lucid dream occurred near the end of my rowdy pulp mill era. After my escape from Royal Roads Military College in Victoria, British Columbia (with an honourable discharge), I worked for just over fourteen years – throughout my twenties and early thirties – as a power engineer at pulp and paper mill power plants in British Columbia, the most westerly province in Canada.

To this day, I still believe that the <u>Angel</u> lucid dream rescued me from dangerous dungeons of sulphur, sweaty high-pressure steam turbine generators (some as big as houses), huge hissing pneumatic control valves, screaming motors, ten story high rumbling black-liquor fired furnaces with red hot smelt spouting into vast dissolving tanks, and the complex piping that leaked toxic chemicals capable of melting human skin upon contact.

Along with many of the lumberjacks out in the vast Canadian forests, plenty of mill workers were injured, maimed and even killed on a regular basis during that period of time in my wild west. As for me, I felt rotten even though I was in the prime of my physical soul's life because I hated my core role in the destruction of our beautiful forests. Owing to the consequences of my own unwholesome attitudes, I was a demon who toiled in the furnaces of hell for over a decade!

The <u>Angel</u> lucid dream banged into existence near the end of my pulp mill era: it was another of those pivotal lucid dreams. When I look back through the dream diaries from that period in my life, my dream memories flood forward. For me, many of the best "times" throughout my twenties and early thirties were experienced in dream worlds. During those years, I went through a phase when I believed that my real-world reality was a stepping stone toward lucid dreaming; my real-life mission was to stay healthy and wealthy enough to make sleeping a priority. I'd sleep for nine to ten hours at a time, usually twelve on my days off from work. But, gee whiz – I was dreaming my life away!

Before the <u>Angel</u> lucid dream took place, I was questioning some of the deeper vibes resonating within my belief system, especially my troubles with lost love, resentment, and my need to show forgiveness; meanwhile, the angel was very beautiful, and I knew her name the instant I saw her – Angela! Although she was perfectly proportioned from head to toe, Angela appeared to be in the order of five meters tall! I remember that her snow-white wings went even higher above her majestic head.

With wings folded, Angela floated down into a deep pit where I stood at the bottom, motionless, and hidden. Similar to a well with a dry bottom, the circular pit was about three to four meters in diameter, lined with brick and mortar, and went for many hundreds of meters.

A light pinch confirmed what I already knew, I was in a dream world. My desire was simply to disappear for a while – this deep pit served my purpose. I brought my calm attention up from the bare earth beneath my feet, gazed aloft, and felt amazed as Angela came floating toward me. Although I wanted some peace and quiet, I welcomed her. She had long curly blonde hair which flowed all around her face and shoulders. And, she had the sunny countenance of an angel! Plus, a soft white light surrounded her, and this radiance lit-up the pit.

When Angela arrived, she held me in a tight hug. Together, we slowly ascended all the way to the top of the pit; then, out into a night sky. Angela was like a winged goddess who had come to the rescue! I felt an emotion that I'd been missing for a long, long while – ever since being embraced by long, loving hugs from my sweet mum when I was a young chap.

After Angela looked down at me and smiled, she asked me to hum on every exhale of breath. Between lengthy spells of humming, I felt myself beginning to channel an idea that I would later describe – following that <u>Soul Saving</u> lucid dream I spoke of at the end of chapter one – as lucid love, for the reason that I recognized a pure and heartfelt energy pouring out of my soul, no strings attached!

Angela's angelic spirit of life fed healthy conscious energy into my dream soul, and while I was loving the present moment, my lucid love fed her outlook with the suitable subconscious energy required to help sustain her presence. I listened closely as she explained how I could give healthier happiness.

Angela spoke softly, "William, oh William, you get trapped into such a hellish place, that presence of mind you're in while working at the pulp mill, all on account of the disagreeable and conflicting energy resonating within your thoughts."

"Oh no!" I cried out, "You mean it's not the pulp mill that's making me feel unhealthy?"

"Absolutely not," came Angela's reply. She had her chin on top of my head – her voice sent tingling vibrations throughout my entire dream body as she said, "Ill health begins with rotten unhappiness deep down inside of your heart. The words you exhale help create the nightmare in which you live. Not only that, your bad attitudes are also absorbed inward and throughout your soul's entire nerve system, which is making you physically sick too."

She was correct. There'd been a recent real-life bout of illness producing a high temperature, sore throat, running nose, headache, dry cough, and muscle pain. Plus, my persistent cough wouldn't go away.

While the two of us slowly ascended higher and higher into the night sky, Angela said, "Next, there're going to be stomach-aches along with much more severe physical illness due to mental health problems eating away at your soul: thinning hair, ongoing rashes which will worsen, muscle and joint problems, pneumonia, even cancer. Your unhealthy attitudes generate rotten energy, which is rotting your heart out. You are indeed turning into a real-life monster!"

I believed her and cried out, "Please help me my sweet angel, what can I do to make things better?"

Angela answered straight away, "Send me some deeper love. You can hum out loud every morning and evening for a mere minute, and when you purr from an attitude connected with a love for life, I'll be with you. Purr in a low tone, one which makes your eardrums vibrate. This works best with earplugs in."

I understood how earplugs could block the ugly noise I'd fed into my real world. By humming out loud while wearing earplugs, I could feel a healing vibration align with the hum of my deeper purr. It was all about going in a deep-purr (deeper) direction!

We floated together for what felt like ages, that angel and I, and all the while, we took turns with our purring. I remember wanting to float with her forever; however, today I understand that ultimately, even such incredible bliss would get boring since "forever" is a never-ending now. Even so, after my eventual jolt back to the real world, and after only a few days of humming with deep-purr purr-pose (deeper purpose) for not even a full minute each morning and evening, my cough went away!

Much later in life, I understood why Angela meant that I needed to feel a love for sharing the present moment – not a crushing greed for possessing an angel. I had to reverse the direction of my thinking in order to give healthy happiness.

This belief in taking a reverse direction in my real world made me cleanup my window of self-awareness in order to get a clearer view of my direction in life. Thanks to earplugs (the soft and foamy type) placed only partially into my ear canals, along with a moderate rate of humming a low "e" note, I could (and still do) get my teeth vibrating in a ticklish way too. Plus, while speaking upbeat words such as joy, love, happy, harmonious, beautiful, and so forth – along with beginning to understand why my real world is similar to another dimension of dreaming – healthy happiness began to feel real!

After connecting my ego with a cleaner, clearer, more wholesome and healthier outlook, something really amazing happened: less than a month after that Angel lucid dream took place, I met a wonderful woman with long curly blonde hair and a radiant smile whose first name turned out to be Angela! I quit my pulp mill job, moved to the southern tip of Vancouver Island, and married her! Even though I thought she was special, I lost her in the end, owing to my recurring spasms of egotism. Since we shared almost two decades of the most amazing union, my being dropped – by a wife whom I believed had the spirit of an angel – pierced my heart and soul with a deep intention to fall into writing self-healing books; a far better path to take than falling upon my own sword!

In retrospect, the <u>Angel</u> lucid dream was trying to teach me to "float" free from my unhappy and unwholesome egotistical mindset; nevertheless,

I did at least learn how a good session of humming is an easy and natural start for some soulful health.

Thinking and speaking from an optimistic tone of voice also helps strengthen an ego's healthier and happier outlook. Once again, an appreciation for how a soul gets affected by certain sounds can channel sound reasoning that'll impress the subconscious mind with healthy, lucidly loving energy. For instance: how many times must you listen to a sad song before deeper thinking kicks in to make you realize that an unhappy mood is limiting your subconscious power to feel a love for the present moment?

An unhappy mood may arrive while you listen to a sad or a proud song because the resonating frequency of energy you "feel" with your ears can be as mind altering as the resonating frequency of energy you send with your voice! While you sing or listen to a joyful song, you can feel good. From wholesome songs about loving the moment… to proud battle tunes of war, what you sing, say, and hear also help shape your subconscious mood. A song is capable of enlivening tones of subconscious energy that a soul can transform into emotion.

As with most broad generalizations, there're usually exceptions, and such is the case with sad music always being an unhealthy experience. Occasionally, those melancholy minor chords may be very beneficial for your psychological and physical wellbeing. Certain sad tones of subconscious energy can strike a chord in almost anyone's heart, and while thinking about a shocking event, your own voice can help you weep out rotten energy.

Shaking and trembling associated with the physical action of sobbing can toss unhealthy subconscious energy frozen from fear. Here comes yet another example of health being ruined by an egotistical thinking mindset because for selfishly proud men and women, whether alone or especially whenever in public, their crying out loud is unacceptable!

Snapping out of egotism occurs when you can focus on an intention to merge your individual outlook with a healthier attitude. This way, an intention to have a healthy attitude helps bring you a healthier soul. A healthier attitude and healthier soul are harmonious with one another and fundamental for developing a really good mood. Lucid love also progresses with a good mood since once again, tossing boredom can be harmonious with loving the present moment. Your ego can help express a healthier presence of mind whether in the real world or in your own lucid dream world.

Resisting ultimate enlightenment, ultimate power, and complete boredom in a lucidly loving way, you can feel healthy and happy. That's why tossing the burden of "ultimate enlightenment" leads to a healthier and happier level of "perfect" enlightenment!

## **Compassionate**

A compassionate outlook goes hand in hand with a balanced mind. Number five of the six special points of view confirms another lifesaving lift into lucid love's deeper subconscious power – the subconscious power to share a strong and positive feeling for being in the present moment.

Without a doubt, you experience a level of self-awareness. That's why you're here! A profound intention to feel compassion for all levels of self-awareness helps save you from those wild waterfalls of egotistical recklessness.

When you're able to feel empathy for another soul's suffering, you're forgiving your deeper self for failure. Viewpoints that flow with guidance from the Lucid Law of Tossing Your Burden mesh with guidance from the Lucid Law of Forgiveness. Tossing a fearful attitude gets plenty of help with a merciful and compassionate viewpoint. For example: if a person commit's a serious crime, you could blame such behaviour on their upbringing, their parents' upbringing, their schooling, their association with teachers, classmates, brothers, sisters, etc. The list goes on and on. A nasty crime comes from more than just one person. An intention to forgive another person for their conscious belief, instead of trying to forgive the person for their ignorant behaviour is a healthier direction for deeper mindfulness.

You're capable of feeling empathy for another's point of view, and this presents another way to love sharing your own perception of the present moment – flaws and all. Another plus point, feeling sympathy for the suffering of your own soul can create a deeper desire to get some control over your own belief! Stepping onward – into the kind of existence that you want to experience includes discovering ways to feel compassionate about wounding backward steps. This way, you can feel thankful for the healing stage.

Flowing with the way a compassionate attitude meshes with guidance from all the lucid laws makes unhappy subconscious rhythms fade away. Your unhealthy behaviour won't repeat thanks to feeling sincere sorrow for anyone's nightmarish outlook. Belief in compassion for everyone's outlook can get you "over with the waterfall" and transcending bad attitudes without denying them.

You may direct deeper subconscious power toward helping, instead of hurting another soul if you can believe that while helping another, you're helping your own real self! A compassionate attitude also summons healthy feedback. Showing sympathy for the suffering of others, often including a desire to help, impresses the subconscious mind with conscious belief that being forgiven feels good, and your soul can also feel good when you forgive.

## Forgiveness For Fearful Feedback

A person is capable of feeling a criminal measure of fear, anger, and hurt. Evil Karmic loops get frozen into the present moment through a soul's fearful, angry, and hurtful feedback. A nightmarish fear of growing old and grey is another example of criminal belief. Hating what you consciously believe to be ugly is as criminal as is the ignorant behaviour returning from unhealthy truth; however, you can feel deeper subconscious power while showing sympathy for belief in ugliness, and you may view old age with compassion.

If an ego resonates with a compassionate outlook, their crumpled old soul is able to return a mood of fearlessness! Since your soul can seem to age very gradually, in an almost imperceptible way, by the time you're very old and crumpled, hair all grey and falling out, half blind, mostly deaf, and having a huge time just getting out of bed, never mind trying to walk, the prospect of your dying isn't going to be so unbelievable as it was when you were young! Because your body's DNA is programmed with plenty of evolutionary wisdom, you're capable of receiving the same compassion that you give.

Tossing fear of old age enables you to comprehend why all souls prepare their shielded levels of self-awareness for a step through "death's door" by aging gradually. When a soul dies, the essence of that soul floats off as a bubble of "evaporated" cosmic energy – a significant type of food for thought – inevitably raining back into life's river of self-awareness.

Comprehending why every soul's cosmic self is the same Great One Dreamer (GOD), you can show compassion for your aged and unattractive looking soul. Being mindful of ideas and understandings arriving from the ways in which all six special viewpoints – and the seven lucid laws – combine with one another, you can impress your subconscious mind with fearless belief about old age and death. You may even live the life of a graceful old soul because grateful attitudes accompany the fearlessness of lucid love!

Subconscious power to channel long-lasting consciousness in the real world arrives when your attitude is harmonious with lucid love. Feeling lucid love's deeper subconscious power tossing fear, anger, hurt, as well as trailing emotions of resentment and guilt helps reveal another major benefit: the sooner belief in compassion can arrive, the quicker you can recover from a shocking event. You need to heal your own broken-hearted soul in order to toss the burden of an unresolved and fearfully shocking emotion being triggered later on.

Some symptoms suffered by shocked souls may include uncontrollable anxiety, fearful flashbacks, panic attacks, insomnia, rage, depression, or any type of criminal mood. Because unhealthy emotional feelings are harmonious with unhealthy outlooks, you can continue to feel physical pain. A shocking fear that's frozen into your soul – from feeling bullied, heartbroken, physically injured, diseased, old and ugly, or even young and ugly – may be hard to step away from. Plenty of people keep their fear, anger, and pain bottled up deep inside. Not only that, if you're suffering from a reincarnated post-traumatic stress disorder, such as the type mentioned in chapter six's bit about reincarnation, you're also suffering from an ancestor's psychological damage due to their having experienced severe emotional shock or distress.

The healthy truth behind belief in compassion can free your soul from fear because you're able to physically grieve whenever you recognize that you're feeling dreadfully lost or upset. When a person is crying, the emotion that they're feeling is free from fear. Weeping releases frozen and semi-frozen criminal energy. Doing yourself justice takes place since healing from any type of broken heart is interconnected with all seven lucid laws. That's because a compassionate attitude is a lucidly loving attitude.

At last, you don't need to fear a past, present, or future heartbreak! Emotional rescue from the unhealthy truth behind belief in losing a loved one can finally arrive after you weep out your feeling of loss from a deeper thinking mindset. Hallelujah! Deeper subconscious power from loving the present moment tosses all fear of heartbreak because lucid love heals!

Giving lucid love – as explained by the Lucid Law of Love – returns lucid love – as explained by the Lucid Boomerang Law – to your time continuum. When you give lucid love, your soul is impressed with deeper subconscious power, the legal power that's capable of healing you from shocking – and criminal – heartbreak. Although an all out sob session releases frozen fear, the healthy energy of a happy mood does the healing. Crying doesn't actually heal. Crying is a more tender form of hurt, a type of subconscious energy that's easier to transform.

While lucid love transforms an emotional heartbreak, you're also capable of washing away the fear flowing from unhealthy DNA. Once again, showing compassion – through the action of trembling and crying from a deeper thinking, real-world presence of mind – enables you to toss cellular memory that's frozen in fear.

Another reason for looking through your own window of self-awareness from a lucidly loving point of view is because just like a boomerang, Karma from your gene pool loops back at you. Through DNA, good or bad fortune can return, thanks to cellular memory. As I mentioned at the finish of chapter six's section on reincarnation, you may suffer from a post-traumatic stress disorder that didn't originate from your individual ego's life experience. But, how do you know if you have criminal cellular memory? From your nightmares of course!

Your soul may bring you an intense emotion from an ancestor. The nightmares you experience during dream worlds – and in the real world – help provide hints and tips for recognizing the sort of rhythmic energy streaming forth from any originating burst of resistance that was inharmonious with loving the present moment. All you need do, when you're ready, is focus in on one criminal mood at a time, and weep it out.

You weep for all your relatives (passed and present), the spirit of all humanity, and the spirit of the cosmic universe when you weep with deeper love pouring from conscious belief in compassion. This way, a subconscious perception of compassion tosses post-traumatic terror! Teardrops transform how you feel because while you weep, you feel no fear – you wash unhealthy energy from your own self-awareness. That's why songs of compassion often contain such axioms as: "Cry me a river."

Compassionate attitudes also involve accepting restitution so that new grudges won't develop. An all out blubbering sob session can make a sincere payment for debts of restitution, releasing you and your DNA from hurtful subconscious memory. Deeper forgiveness takes place when you view "blundering" conscious and subconscious energy with compassion; then, bad Karma can finally stop looping back!

A profound intention to show compassion for all levels of self-awareness helps you transcend fear. When you stop blaming people, animals, events, or anything else for not being the way they should be, you can stop taking selfish attitudes so seriously. Instead of trying to love somebody from a greedy and egotistical point of view, an intention to share a love for the present moment – with another soul (or souls) – is another way to give lucid love.

## Trustful

This sixth special viewpoint begins with an intention to trust that similar to a dream world, the real world is part of a multidimensional mind – exciting stuff! Such trust enables conscious belief that no matter how old, ugly, sick, or beautiful you may appear to be, making your real-world reality feel like a healthy dream can happen within a heartbeat!

Even if you're fit and strong, you can still benefit from trusting in a healthy truth behind the meaning of your life. For example: you may certainly trust that your attitudes have effects. That's why, through the deeper subconscious power you get from feeling a present mood that you can love, unhealthy truths transform. The real reason why lucid love amplifies healthy energy during a lucid dream world and in the real world is because while you're loving the present moment, good things happen – automatically. When you feel good, good things really can happen without your having to consciously micromanage everything.

As explained in chapter three, the lucid laws are a guiding force – just like the laws of gravity and the laws of electricity. To harness the power of gravity, electricity, the cosmic mind, and your own mind, you need to balance conscious and subconscious energy. Understanding the way that the seven lucid laws mesh enables you to trust in the cumulative power of all energy! The lucid laws are ideas helping to guide a person into feeling happiness by way of establishing conscious belief in all levels of self-awareness being the present moment, as well as being the essence of a cosmic mind.

We all need courage in order to change a belief. Then again, by trusting in the greater power of deeper thinking, you may dare to exercise some real bravery – toss old fear, anger, and hurt. This way, you can consciously believe in a harmoniously joyful, lucidly loving, and delightfully surprising world view!

Hateful and angry attitudes don't contribute to an existence that feels good. A lucidly loving outlook lets you view violent or aggressive acts with the intention of surviving in an energy consuming food chain instead of viewing them as an offence to your ego. Trusting that a deeper, real-life cosmic self is a whole dreaming mind can nourish kinder moods that feel good, whereas fearful, angry, or hurtful attitudes feed those nightmarish moods that make your present moment feel like crap.

You're capable of bridging into a deeper thinking, real-life presence of mind by trusting that your real-life reality is similar to another dimension of dreaming. While surviving in an energy consuming food chain, a deeper trust in your real self being cosmic can get you in harmony with how you want to feel.

Ignoring lucid love's deeper power to automatically manage subconscious energy – in a healthy way – can make way for a very slippery slope, a direction where a slide into mayhem can take place on account of egotism taking offence to a hungry, real-world reality. Hunger is a powerful reminder about why every soul must be fed with more than just a hope for happiness. Trying to get gloriously high on mere hope for happiness may sound silly, but such short-sightedness can feed a world of self-awareness with more fear, anger, and hurt; however, having hope is handy for recognizing that you aren't getting your needs met.

Trying to get gloriously high on a trust in lucid love may also sound silly, but such farsightedness can feed a world of self-awareness with harmonious joy, lucid love, and delightful surprise!

CHAPTER TEN

# A QUICK REVIEW OF LUCID LAW

**W**hy are you alive, and who really cares? Why do you have to suffer? Who and what is God? Where does a belief in God come from? How can you possibly describe a meaningful point to life? All of these profound questions have been answered in useful, thankful, respectful, healthy, compassionate, and trustful ways because we've been flowing in a lucidly loving direction of thought. So way to go, you've made it! Welcome to a whole new world view of your present moment. And, welcome to a deeper thinking, more powerful, real-world presence of mind!

Who in their right mind can gain a meaningful and self empowering view on the significance of a single human life flowing in the vastness of the universe, let alone the depth of eternity? You can! Lucid dreaming, lucid awareness, and Lucid Law enable you to discover a meaningful, self empowering, and clearer view on deeper self-definition. Basically, a cosmic self views the vastness of an instantaneous "here" and "now" reality from as many shielded windows of self-awareness as there are dream souls and real-world souls, all at the same time!

Along with deeper self-definition, caring about the present moment brings an unconventional concept of time. Whenever you experience a gloomy world view, you're not loving your present moment. You can get some deeper subconscious power to love your present moment and feel long-lasting, healthy happiness when you understand the important ideas pouring from lucid dreaming, lucid awareness, and Lucid Law.

All seven lucid laws intertwine with the six special points of view described in chapter nine. Ignoring the six special points of view (useful, thankful, respectful, healthy, compassionate, and trusting) is dangerous since they're as lawful as legal acts can be. In every legal court of law, whatever nasty thing you've said or done can be held against you. By the same ruling, whatever nice thing you've said or done can be used to help you. And it's the same deal with Lucid Law.

The lucid laws take you along a new path of "perfect" enlightenment because although your egotism gets blown away, your ego strengthens with healthy truth behind belief in a different level of self-definition. Being mindful of "perfect" enlightenment empowers your ego by stepping you onward, where the effects of healthy truth may be felt deep down in the heart of it all – the "heart" of your soul.

## The Lucid Law Of Love

A lucidly loving outlook is a perfect type of enlightenment thanks to a healthy ego guarding you from that nemesis of ultimate enlightenment – a state of never-ending boredom. A healthy ego also exemplifies a paradox: you express an individual level of self-awareness, yet, you're also linked with a deeper, cosmic self. Healthy truth behind the Lucid Law of Love is all about the idea that giving lucid love makes your present moment "feel" beautiful. Just like a dream world, the real world may feel beautiful or ugly, depending upon your subconscious mood. This way, your subconscious mind channels a sensational dimension of reality! A person may sense that their existence is objective because a physical universe seems to be based on facts rather than thoughts, opinions, or feelings. That's how a seemingly individual presence of mind is protected from ultimate power, ultimate enlightenment, and total boredom.

The Lucid Law of Love is all about a lucidly loving attitude being a perfect level of enlightenment because such an outlook impresses your soul with a healthy, lucidly loving mood. Subconscious power becomes controllable in a healthy way – while lucid love is impressed upon your subconscious mind. Similar to a long-lasting lucid dream world, feeling long-lasting lucid love provides more and more subconscious power for you to enjoy a healthy, real-world existence. In other words, for the love of GOD, step into a lucidly loving mood and save your soul!

Insight into the Lucid Law of Love can also help to transform an egotistical level of self-awareness. It's important to toss egotism before your soul dies because when your ego passes through death's door, conscious and subconscious energy are going to have an effect on the transformation of your mind. Balanced mind, healthy transformation!

Discovering that your real self is a cosmic dreamer, you can impress your subconscious mind in safe and wholesome ways. The reason you're safe is because giving lucid love returns a healthy present moment – a wholesome presence of mind that keeps you free from evil attitudes. What's more, you may step into a lucidly loving presence of mind in a heartbeat since a lucidly loving attitude is only a thought away. That's why, through a more transparent window of self-awareness, you're "wider" awake and feeling great!

Resonating within every seemingly individual soul, a cosmic dreamer experiences different outlooks in order to feel "new" life. A shielded level of self-awareness defines the reason for every soul's existence. When you can consciously believe that your soul channels a greater dreaming self, your physical body can feel deeper happiness.

If your ego implodes due to a shocked, hardened, and unhealthy world view, you're capable of some major disappointment caused by your unhealthy truths. Disillusionment denies conscious belief that every soul channels the same deeper self-awareness; then, egotistical belief that you're separate and superior returns a fear of inferiority and isolation.

Denying yourself a clear intention to stir up some lucid love for whatever present moment you're experiencing, you can completely forget about who you really are. If you believe that existence is hurtful instead of realizing that your perception of existence is what truly hurts, your disapproving attitudes, words, and behaviours also make your dream worlds feel hurtful. Even though you may want to change an unhealthy outlook, the same old nasty moods can keep looping back at you. That's because first of all, you need to change your belief in self-definition.

## The Lucid Law Of Resistance

Linking with a belief in your real self being a dreaming mind, you can trust that you are time, space, and all levels of self-awareness – instantaneously. This way, you can be all over the Lucid Law of Resistance! Arriving hand over fist with a lucidly loving presence of mind, you can resist boredom in healthy ways.

Bringing conscious and subconscious energy into balance answers how the Lucid Law of Resistance has meaning. There's a balance between the "good" of a little boredom and the "evil" of complete boredom. Less resistive conscious energy enables calmness and control. With calmness and control, you may comprehend how an individual level of self-awareness here in the real world is similar to an individual level of self-awareness in a dream world. Individualism is an imaginative illusion that feels real, thanks to physical resistance. Every physical soul is here to resist ultimate enlightenment because such a deep level of self-awareness is the pathway to oblivion from boredom.

A totally bored spirit of life is an example of an unbalanced mind. Through guidance from the Lucid Law of Resistance, you can resist the imbalance of too much subconscious control and a boring outlook. Resisting boredom in healthy ways also lights up the unconventional view that a declaration of love for another soul, instead of a declaration to share a love for another level of the same present moment, can unbalance your mind!

A deeper thinking intention to share a love for life – with another soul – returns a feel for lucid love. Feeling lucid love is different from feeling a desire and longing for ownership over another soul. That's because lucid love is given… not taken.

A delightfully surprising state of healthy lust for a mate usually begins with a fresh honeymoon phase. This is a phase when life can feel so great that your entire world may look and feel very beautiful because lust can feel harmoniously joyful! Problems arrive when you demand to own the physical body you're lusting for – instead of intending to share an especially special level of self-awareness. Belief in owning another soul is similar to demanding satisfaction from feeding your subconscious hunger with unhealthy conscious energy. Lucid love is healthy food for thought whereas egotistical greed can be bitter-sweet for an unthinking subconscious hunger to live.

If you can understand the healthier idea of loving to share your present moment with the person whom you want to get intimate with, instead of wanting to eat the person alive, your own subconscious soul can steer you clear of bad Karma from unhealthy, yet, super sweet thoughts of total control. Romance fades with the inevitable boredom of ultimate possession; the honeymoon phase ends, and the present moment may not seem so great anymore. Feeling a loss of lust owing to the burden of boredom invites an unhealthy attitude.

Jealousy is another way to ease the burden of a boring relationship, but jealousy is inharmonious with the way most people want to feel. For one thing, perhaps your partner might really feel new lustful desire for another soul! With such a disconnect, your thoughts may impress your soul with a conscious belief in heartbreak.

A conscious desire for ultimate possession of another soul puts a huge burden on the subconscious mind. That's because heartbreak is inevitable. Plus, heartbreak can churn out angry thoughts, words, and conduct, bringing death to a romantic present moment. Along with burdening belief in heartbreak, your subconscious mind automatically pressures your ego by making you feel inharmonious with a deeper love for your own presence. Your life's path can continue to get even more contorted as the same sort of broken-hearted emotions keep flying back at you. And there's no getting away; there can appear to be no freedom.

Demanding that love be about a perception of ownership, instead of being about a perception of deeper self-awareness, you can be hit hard again and again with the loss of romance. Jealousy isn't a good direction to take because owing to the fear of your partner desiring another soul, the shocking reality of such truth can hurt so bad that you may be traumatized by the ordeal!

Expressing a lucidly loving resistance to heartbreak helps you survive and evolve – you're not stuck with inflexible attitudes. If your partner wants to share their present moment with somebody else, you don't have to resist inharmoniously… you can toss an egotistical outlook. You may feel empty for a while, but when you purposely toss selfishness and greed by weeping with the deeper truth behind belief in forgiveness, you can heal.

Forgiveness for your own soul no longer being the object of your ex's desire returns balance to your presence of mind; then, broken-hearted feelings stop looping back. The present moment includes your ex's presence of mind; a healthy way to achieve long-lasting happiness is to share a lucidly loving outlook with an ex – if there's no escaping their presence!

If you feel unhappy, your own soul is punishing you by making your present moment bring about the reality of your own rotten attitude. A ruling behind the Lucid Law of Resistance is that unhealthy resistance to boredom can really hurt! This is why people suffer. For example: after a burst of resentful anger coming from belief in an injustice, you may ask why you couldn't stay in a permanent state of joy? Once happiness is set in motion, you might think that the good mood should be ceaseless since a ruling of the Lucid Boomerang Law is that whatever you say or do loops back at you; however, I'm sure you can agree that for most folks, happiness doesn't seem to fly for very long.

## The Lucid Boomerang Law

The reason happiness isn't self-perpetuating for most folks is because unhealthy happiness disconnects a human soul from deeper self-definition. The Lucid Boomerang Law is all about thoughts, words, and actions returning a deeper definition of the present moment. So, one way or another, self-definition has an effect on your world view.

Winning at gambling on card games is an example of unhealthy happiness being inharmonious with a long-term good mood because in order to win, others must lose. When you realize that "others" also help define your present moment, you may understand why you can't really win if they lose! By the same token, they can't really win if you lose! That's because everyone is the same self!

Happiness that's harmonious with selfishness and greed takes you in a direction that won't maintain such unhealthy happiness since the selfish mood you've enlivened distorts the definition of happiness. Honest intention to satisfy a selfishly greedy and superior outlook is destined to generate fear, anger, and hurt in the long run. The Lucid Boomerang Law parallels a Biblical Law of destiny – according to Hindu and Buddhist religion, the quality of a person's current and future life is determined by that person's behaviour in this and previous lives.

As explained in chapter six, science reveals why reincarnation may be more accurately understood as subconscious memory being passed down through a gene pool. This category of memory instructs your soul's development with the subconscious power coming from your own soul's DNA (deoxyribonucleic acid). Subconscious memory of shock and trauma can sour any soul. Severe subconscious memory sets the stage for sinister fate to fly back at you, just like a nightmarish boomerang hitting you in the face because you didn't see it coming!

Whether you or an ancestor flew into a really hurtful outlook from an evil twist of fate, until the original impression of severe hurtfulness can be forgiven, your subconscious mind is going to make you keep on suffering. The Lucid Boomerang Law also reveals that similar to a dream world, the real world spins with healthy and unhealthy happiness. Another difference between good and evil is all about healthy and unhealthy truth behind belief in happiness because for one thing, an evil mood eventually loops back from unhealthy perception.

Unhealthy subconscious memory can antagonize a person's outlook; a good mood may go off course as you plunge in a direction that's capable of channelling an evil attitude. In the case of reincarnating bad Karma, what's actually happening is that an antagonized outlook keeps flying back from an ancestor's traumatized soul.

Understanding why the Lucid Boomerang Law's guiding power meshes with a show of compassion for the presence of self-awareness, you can transform bad Karma. That's because you can toss a Karmic boomerang in a lucidly loving direction! The healthy truth behind a belief in your real-world reality being related to the space-time continuum of a dream world enables you to step out of bad Karmic loops by channelling your thoughts, words, and actions through a compassionate point of view.

The "Butterfly Effect" is another illustration of the Lucid Boomerang Law. That the tiny breeze made by a butterfly's fluttering wings can have an effect on the weather also suggests that tiny cues can have an effect the way you weather life, for instance, a butterfly can also be a quantum cue for triggering conscious belief in beauty flying free. Beauty – in the eye of the beholder – can return a crushing desire for ownership.

Watching a butterfly fly free before a crush of desire to own such beauty fades, selfishness and greed might make you want to hunt down the butterfly and own it! After mounting the butterfly's soul in a glass case or in some sort of a butterfly book, such belief in beauty still fades because eventually, staring at a dead butterfly can feel hugely boring.

When you give lucid love, you get the kind of deeper subconscious power that makes sharing your present moment feel beautiful. Since you may honestly believe this new idea that your real self is a present space-time continuum, you may sense the deeper beauty within a healthier mood. By giving lucid love, you can take ownership of a healthier way to weather life; loving to share the present moment with another soul balances long-term happiness.

## The Lucid Law Of Forgiveness

Healthier subconscious energy emerges from understanding a basic idea behind the Lucid Law of Forgiveness: subconscious memory flies back at you with gravitational waves of streaming rhythm. When you intend to transform unhealthy subconscious memory (no matter how bitter-sweet), your ego can go in a healthier direction. This way, you may forgive your own subconscious mind for fearful feedback.

Suffering in a world of energy eating souls arrives through unhealthy patterns of words, thoughts, and behaviours. Using the Lucid Law of Forgiveness to illustrate this hugely important point about the measurable benefit you get from transforming unhealthy subconscious memory helps direct your own ego toward a more forgiving outlook. While you forgive yourself for feeling unhappy, you're forgiving your cosmic mind for going down paths of selfishness and greed. Thanks to a forgiving attitude, you can turn yourself around!

Forgiveness for a selfish outlook goes hand in hand with loving to share the present moment. Instead of holding a grudge, holding onto the important understandings from the Lucid Law of Forgiveness can help guide you into deeper self-definition and impress your soul with a different feel for life. When your subconscious mind accepts the Lucid Law of Forgiveness as being a valid direction for self-definition, lucid love's deeper subconscious power enables you to feel the forgiveness that you give.

Calm, warm, and smooth flowing conscious energy that's channelled to life by your feeling mercy makes it possible for you to feel good when you're facing what would otherwise be judged as an adversity. In chapter nine there was some discussion about how you might age gracefully through a compassionate point of view. Also of incredible consequence, now that you know how to heal from your loss of a partner, family member, friend, or pet in a natural and forgiving way, you know that you're safe to keep on loving your present moment.

An unforgiving attitude can have you being ruled by a lot more than just the crappy consequences accompanying a belief in your superiority. Criticizing another for their ignorant mistakes makes inferiority become real for you. If you refuse to forgive anyone, anything, or even your own soul for not being good enough, your ego can also judge your own inferiority from an imploded, cold-hearted, and ugly point of view. Flowing with an evil attitude makes your soul return a sickening world view of shocking insanity!

## The Lucid Law Of Belief

Guiding your soul into a mood that's harmonious with feeling unconditional love for the One present moment gets you some deeper subconscious power to control your destiny because you're also impressing your cosmic soul with a belief in lucid love. The Lucid Law of Belief is about understanding the idea that if you merely expect a healthier mood to bring you a healthier outlook, your ego can evolve.

Whether or not your belief in self-definition is what you want it to be, such thought feels real. At hand is another perfect example for you to realize why your conscious belief has a huge effect on how you feel: a medical doctor's blue pill, which is only an innocent food capsule (or tablet) made blue by food colouring, can sometimes cure a patient's illness! The placebo is a preparation containing no medicine, but is given for positive effects. Well known in medical circles, the "Placebo Effect" is an example of active trust rather than idle hope.

You can also cure illness with subconscious power coming from trusting in healthy truth behind the Lucid Law of Belief. That's because deeper subconscious power from a cosmic universe made you in the first place! The power of your subconscious mind can heal you, if you let it. Belief in lucid love unlocks healthy subconscious energy to heal your physical body – automatically.

The Lucid Law of Belief also reveals why, for some folks, whether it be good or bad, luck feels real. Belief that a cosmic soul is the "physical" universe can free you from luck having power over your real-life soul. You don't need to believe in luck in order to feel healthy happiness. You're capable of feeling healthier moods in dreams and in the real world while showing respect for the idea that good fortune gets channelled by Karma-loops. Good fortune comes from healthy belief being impressed upon the subconscious mind, and good Karma loops back like a boomerang.

While in a lucid dream world, there's no sense in believing that good fortune comes from a different source than evil fortune, even though good and evil oppose one another. As with good and evil, love and hate are opposites here in the real world too. You may consciously believe that your lovely times are your good times, whereas an evil attitude eventually feels hate all of the time. The idea behind the Lucid Law of Belief is to guide subconscious energy into making good times last longer.

Then again, if you ignore the Lucid Law of Belief's guidance to take your subconscious mind in a lucidly loving direction, you're capable of abusing your subconscious power. By expecting your existence to be crappy, you might get some surprises, but they won't feel healthy. Yet, to be caught unawares, attacked, or surprised in any disastrous way, you still shield your deeper self from eternal boredom by way of your grim belief in a nightmarish present moment being real!

The Lucid Law of Belief is also about realizing that the real-world space-time continuum is a dimension of universal self-awareness. The realization that a present moment arrived with a cosmic mind banging real-life reality into existence is a healthy way to channel conscious belief in a deeper self being present in the fabric of all subconscious energy. Such belief can impress your subconscious mind with a loving feel for a universal presence – a real-world present moment.

Being present and in the moment while at the same time believing in a lucidly loving link with a deeper, more powerful real-world presence of mind, you can strengthen the health of your own soul. You get a stronger and healthier real-world soul because conscious belief that a deeper point to real-world existence is all about unburdening everyone's heaviest load – eternal boredom – gives you a really important reason to live!

## The Lucid Law Of Living In The Now

Deeper connection with the present moment can get your soul to feel a long-lasting presence of harmonious joy. The Lucid Law of Living in the Now is all about a point of view that's harmonious with loving the "now". This Lucid Law provides sound reasoning for the old saying that "more important than reaching a destination, a joyful journey with life – while it's happening – matters most."

Once again, the Lucid Law of Living in the Now is different from the Lucid Law of Love because the Lucid Law of Love is all about giving deeper love: it's about how you can feel so healthy, beautiful, and happy by loving to be present. The Lucid Law of Living in the Now is about understanding why a present moment for a dream world arrives from the subconscious mind banging a new dimension of self-awareness into existence.

By realizing that "Dreamtime" is self-awareness, you can connect ever-more closely with belief that the real-world time continuum is self-awareness. Believing that the real world parallels a dimension of dreaming helps you redefine self-awareness. Self-awareness may be redefined as a cosmic presence of mind being the real universe – a real-life space-time continuum. That's why you may consciously believe that your purpose in life is to resist the nemesis of ultimate enlightenment – eternal boredom.

Similar to everyone as well as everything in a dream world, everyone as well as everything in the real world also connect an instantaneous now. Consciously believing that your present moment banged into existence from the subconscious power of a cosmic mind can bring you courage to trust that your real self is eternal. By understanding why your real spirit of life includes all individual levels of conscious and subconscious energy, all at once, your deeper thinking mindset can control deeper subconscious power by flowing with an attitude that loves the present moment!

A section in chapter seven (A Paradox Of Self-awareness) also asks where the cosmic self comes from. A paradoxical answer arrives by comparing flowing streams and rivers of water with flowing streams and rivers of life. That's because all life forms flow with an awareness of the present moment. An individual level of human consciousness may be thought of as akin to one droplet in a universal flow of self-awareness. The same way a droplet can't be the flow even though the flow is every droplet, you can't be the Great One Dreamer even though this GOD is you!

Once more, here's the paradox: just as a greater flow of water arrives from a connection with more water droplets, a greater presence of mind arrives from a connection with more individual levels of conscious and subconscious self-awareness; however, even though a river is each water droplet, a droplet is not the river. Similarly, a level of ego conscious can't be the river of life. A presence of mind – the one present moment – lives dream worlds and the real world from shallower, shielded points of view. Paradoxically, similar to how a dream world unfolds, a real-world time continuum unfolds to make a cosmic level of self-awareness feel individual, new, and alive!

While a lucidly loving world view lights up an idea that a cosmic self is the One who designs and lives your real-world reality, you may appreciate why, during everyone's idea of a here and now dimension of reality, now's the time to live! Worry over an ugly past and fear of an even uglier future can disconnect you from living in the "now". The Lucid Law of Living in the Now helps bring you deeper power to love being part of the present moment instead of believing to be apart from the present moment.

Belief in being apart from the present moment goes against guidance from the Lucid Law of Living in the Now because denying a loving connection with your present moment can impress your subconscious mind with unhappiness. While flowing with a spirit of unhappiness, you can bring real-world nightmares into existence! The same way a level of self-awareness within a dream world can have an effect on the way the dream world flows, a level of self-awareness within the real world can have an effect on the way the real world flows.

Loving the present moment makes celebrating the past and trusting in a happy future easy. Loving your own presence of mind also makes healthy happiness flow with renewed conscious and subconscious energy. This way, you can continue to consciously believe that parallel to a dream world space-time continuum being a presence of mind, the real-world space-time continuum is a presence of mind!

You stay in tune with the Lucid Law of Living in the Now while giving thanks for having a presence of mind. Such thankfulness can also protect your orb of ego conscious from being consumed by a beastly presence of mind after your own soul's death because while giving thanks for the idea that "now" is a beautiful moment, your orb of ego conscious is food for healthier thought – a more loving present moment.

If your surroundings aren't pleasing, you might want to give yourself a light pinch and send your lucid love back (Front To Back Thinking) to the present moment – then in an instant, your window of self-awareness can brighten. Merely open your mind, contemplate, and remember why all seemingly individual souls channel the same self. There's an inconspicuous equality to every living entity because every One of us streams within the same cosmic mind.

## **The Lucid Law Of Tossing Your Burden**

Along with responsibility to love your presence of mind, the idea behind the Lucid Law of Tossing Your Burden helps lighten the load. Living proof is already here! As I mentioned in chapter three, thanks to personal computers and cell phones, OMG (Oh… My… GOD) gets sent worldwide in text messages, blogs, tweets, e-mails, and regular mail.

If you pay attention to your present moment, you can hear lots of people calling out, "Oh My GOD!" The real intention behind such an interjection is to jolt everyone back into being more aware of the present moment! Such an interjection is a jolting phrase making you instantly aware of how real your life can feel because OMG has no other meaning for most folks! There's intention behind this edgy comment since it tosses the greatest burden of all time – boredom.

By intending to toss the burden of boredom in healthy ways, so as to celebrate life with nicer surprises, you can! Best of all, by believing that real-life reality parallels a dimension of dream reality, you can toss fear of death. As described in chapter nine, guidance from the Lucid Law of Tossing Your Burden floats and buoys six lucidly loving points of view to help toss burdening egotism: useful, thankful, respectful, healthy, compassionate, and trusting.

## A Fun-loving Finish!

Your mind fabricates a dream world, making you feel real while you're there. A cosmic mind fabricates the real world, making you feel real while you're here – my concluding parallel. That's why you're capable of feeling deeper love for the present moment – no matter who or where you are!

While giving lucid love, you get enough conscious control over your own subconscious power to automatically make a belief in healthy truth feel real. Because your ego flows with a subconscious mood, you're capable of creating a flow of truer love. Where else could a flow of truelove come from? Nowhere else because the same as with all dimensions of dream reality, love is only as real as you can imagine it to be.

The magic of imagination rests in the palms of all hands, and even with all hands on deck, everyone is the "Captain and Crew" of their own direction in life. You can hum and purr with the healthy truth that your direction in life is significant and worthy because deep-purr purr-pose (deeper purpose) is to toss boredom by way of your individual point of view. An ancient nursery rhyme points the way for you to keep on humming up lucid love…

> Row, row, row your boat
> gently down the stream
> merrily, merrily, merrily,
> life is but a dream!

www.ingramcontent.com/pod-product-compliance
Lightning Source LLC
LaVergne TN
LVHW041636060526
838200LV00040B/1586